T0281320

Mothers in Medicine

Katherine Chretien
Editor

Mothers in Medicine

Career, Practice, and Life Lessons Learned

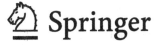 Springer

Editor
Katherine Chretien, MD
Assistant Dean for Student Affairs and Associate Professor of Medicine
George Washington University School of Medicine and Health Sciences
Washington, DC, USA

ISBN 978-3-319-68027-9   ISBN 978-3-319-68028-6   (eBook)
https://doi.org/10.1007/978-3-319-68028-6

Library of Congress Control Number: 2017958349

Printed on acid-free paper

This Springer imprint is published by Springer Nature
The registered company is Springer International Publishing AG
The registered company address is: Gewerbestrasse 11, 6330 Cham, Switzerland

For Jolie, Jean-Luc, Pascal, and Jean-Paul

Foreword

Much of medical school orientation was a blur. But there is one presentation that I remember so clearly, even all these years later. A stern-looking geneticist told us that she and her husband wanted to have children while they were in medical school. But life was too hectic, so they decided to wait until they graduated. But then they were in residency and things were way too crazy, so they decided to wait until fellowship. But research overwhelmed them, so they decided to wait until they were attendings.

You probably know where this story is going. When they were finally safely ensconced as attendings, they decided to start their family and they were not able to conceive. The moral was, clearly, don't wait. But that's not the message that I took from this presentation. As a newbie medical student about to plunge into an MD-PhD program that seemed to have no end in sight, my take-home was, "Shit, that stuff is way too complicated and way too scary. I'm avoiding it at all costs!"

Despite the geneticist's warning to us, though, almost no one had children during medical school and residency. Other than a few orthodox Jewish couples, I didn't see anyone pregnant during my training.

Fast forward two decades when I was now an attending. The medical ward was practically a maternity ward! Everyone was pregnant—residents, fellows, students. I was blown away, but I was also impressed. People were choosing to have kids at whatever time was the right time for them, and they'd figure out the details later.

For me, the right time had turned out to be when I was a new attending. In fact I was early in my second pregnancy when I was making rounds with a new team one July. I noticed that the third-year medical student was quite noticeably pregnant. Rounds were long, and it was hot, so I offered to let her sit down. I thought I'd be able to offer my great wisdom, both as an attending and as someone who had been through the pregnancy-childbirth-daycare ordeal before. She smiled and shrugged off my offers of help. "It's okay," she said. "I have triplets at home, so this is nothing."

That's when I realized that we really *had* come a long way. Medical training was no longer the seventh circle of hell that you had to get safely behind you before you could start your life. It *was* your life, and you could make choices about what you did and didn't want to include in that life.

I don't kid myself that these vaunted choices aren't acutely framed by finances, family support, workplace support, and random chance. But the idea that you were actually living during those years, not just biding time until you could make your debut as a bonafide adult, was a radical conclusion. And it applied not just to having children but to all aspects of life.

A medical classmate of mine confided in me that he'd always wanted to play the saxophone. There was clearly no time for music lessons during medical school, but he realized that if there was no time during medical school, there certainly wouldn't be any time in residency or fellowship. He didn't want to wait a decade to see if he actually liked the sax, and so he scraped up time to play (usually in lieu of meals). He ultimately concluded that it was really only the low mournful notes of the saxophone that appealed to him, so he switched to cello.

His story stuck with me for years as I took up the cello in mid-attendinghood. I now had three kids and a full-time academic job, plus a writing career. I certainly had no time for cello lessons. But until when, exactly, could I put this off: Emeritus? Retirement? Nursing home? Post-mortem?

And so I just did it—bought the cello and signed up for lessons. I fell in love and the cello has become an essential part of my life. I don't miss my lessons *or* practice unless someone is actively hemorrhaging or in status epilepticus—patients or family! It's grown now to the point where we've formed a string quartet that practices in the hospital on Thursday nights after my evening clinic session.

Having children, pursing music, taking up writing—these are all things that have come to define how I live. There are still only 24 hours in the day, of course, so we all have to prioritize and inevitably give some things up. I'll confess that my medical journals pile up in the bathroom unread and that I've never seen a single TV series after "ER." My children remain eternally embarrassed that I know nothing of pop culture and they don't want to be seen in the presence of my thrift-shop clothes or 10-year-old shoes. They've resigned themselves to the fact that we have only three different dinners, and these have been in rotation for 15 years, with little prospect of changing in the next 15 years. Those are the trade-offs I've chosen to make to create a livable life for me. Every person will figure out their own trade-offs.

The experiences of those who've contributed to "Mothers in Medicine" are frustrating, rewarding, agonizing, creative, exhausting, and illuminating. They are as varied as the individual personality types multiplied by the different medical specialties multiplied by the range of resources available. What they have in common, though, is the recognition that life is lived in real time.

We in medicine are inculcated in the culture of deferred enjoyment, of sacrificing our lives now for some distant rose-colored, board-certified future. But here's the breaking news: No chapter with unlimited time and resources is ever going to magically open up in our lives. No fairy godmother will miraculously graft 8 hours onto your day or stock your house with groceries or impress the 16 kinds of vasculitis into your cingulate gyrus.

Postponing "until" turns out to be a futile exercise in continually moving the goalposts northward. At some point, we all have to accept that we are living in the here and now. Our life is not a staging ground for the real life that starts at some undefined moment in the future. What we have is what we have.

I admit that this could be a depressing thought, especially if you are working a 36-hour shift right now and sleeping in a call room that smells like an adolescent's socks. However, shedding the burden of "waiting until" could also be liberating.

I encourage all of us to accept that our life—warts and all—is now. At the very least, this gives us an honest knowledge of what our life is. And it is certainly easier to plan around an imperfect reality than around some fuzzy future idyll, which may or may not ultimately bear any resemblance to what we've been counting on.

"Carpe diem" may be an old chestnut. But the current diem is the only diem we have, certainly the only one we know. It pays for us to choose what we want to do in this diem. If we leave everything to a future diem, someone else—or some other circumstance—may end up making those choices for us. The music is starting now.

New York University School of Medicine   Danielle Ofri, MD, PhD
New York, NY

Preface

Mothers in Medicine is a group blog by physician mothers, writing about the unique challenges and joys of tending to two distinct patient populations, both of whom can be quite demanding. We are on call every. single. day.

-www.mothersinmedicine.com

On a Friday night in May 2008, my husband and I were driving back home to D.C. after an event. I had recently published an essay "Paying at the Pump" that chronicled my experience as a new mother back at work [1], juggling pumping and my clinical practice. This meant developing an unhealthy relationship with my breast pump and a certain level of mania. I wrote about that time lovingly and with humor, even though it wasn't nearly as lovely or funny *at the time*. It was often chaotic, trying, and sometimes very lonely.

After the piece was published, my inbox exploded with emails from men and women from around the country, thanking me for writing about a topic they felt was critical but underrepresented in the medical sphere. The outpouring convinced me that we needed more of these stories shared—messy, imperfect stories of women and motherhood and medicine.

I was telling my husband, also a physician, about some of those responses in the car that night when I had an idea. "What about a group blog of physician mothers telling their stories, forming an online community of support?"

We talked through what it might look like. At the time, I wrote a personal blog and contributed to several other blogs. I thought about people I knew from the blogging world who were physician moms. By the time we reached our home, I had already formed the email message in my mind to prospective writers. On Saturday, I sent emails out, some to women I had never talked to or interacted with before but who wrote blogs that I admired. By Sunday, I had already received an enthusiastic "Yes!" from everyone I reached out to. Those women signed on to be the first regular contributors of the group blog, taking a huge leap of faith along with me. That weekend, Mothers in Medicine was born.

The first post was published on May 26, 2008.

"While in high school, I heard that some store managers were suspicious of teens due to shoplifting incidents. Afterwards, I felt guilty whenever just browsing a store with managers in view. I had no reason to feel guilty. I didn't have sticky fingers. But, somehow, I had already learned to internalize projected judgments of others onto myself.

I get the same slinking feeling whenever I'm leaving work on the early side, taking advantage of getting all of my work done early to get home to spend more time with my children while they're still awake. Even if I plan to continue doing work after they go to bed, I feel like a shadowy criminal trying to get away with something.

I dread running into people who may look at me with all of my bags and then glance down at their watch. I dread running into a supervisor.

It doesn't matter if I'm incredibly efficient and productive during my time at work. Or if I've worked through lunch scarfing down a sandwich in between keystrokes on the computer. It's what the hands on the clock read when I'm leaving the building that determine my innocence."

—KC, "Criminal," May 26, 2008

From the beginning, my goal of Mothers in Medicine (or MiM affectionately in short) has been to support women navigating motherhood and a career in medicine through the open sharing of our stories. We have had dozens of women who have contributed to the blog as regular contributors, and perhaps hundreds have written guest posts or sent in "MiM Mail" for advice. Regular contributors have spanned an array of specialties and now also include medical students and residents. Writers have shared their vulnerabilities, triumphs, observations, joys, and tragedies over the years to a growing community of readers throughout the world. I have often referred to MiM as a labor of love; we all write and support the site on a voluntary basis. When a reader writes in to say that she only survived medical school or residency by reading our blog or that another reader decided to pursue a career in medicine because of it, it reminds us all of the power of a freely accessible forum of support, that our stories are important.

This book is a natural extension of MiM and aligned with our mission of supporting all mothers in medicine, current and future. In the chapters ahead, our authors, some longtime MiM writers, some new, share insights and wisdom gleaned from their own personal experience as well as drawn from the over 1500 posts and thousands of comments from the community posted to the blog to date on key topics that mothers in medicine face. Selected post excerpts and reader comments are sprinkled throughout the chapters. Chapter 1 starts us off with reflections on the initial considerations when choosing (or being chosen) to become a mother in medicine. The final chapter, "Question and Answer," synthesizes the collective wisdom shared on the blog in response to the most commonly asked questions we have received over the years. And in between, our authors discuss everything from having children during medical training, to work-life balance, to navigating life challenges such as divorce, to occupational hazards for the mother in medicine. The chapters do not have to be read in order as readers may be in different stages of their career and motherhood and mentorship; readers can pick and choose as appropriate.

A colleague once asked me, "Why do you share?" It was a general question, an innocent question, asked after he heard about Mothers in Medicine and some of the personal stories I have shared in the medical storytelling space. That question went to the heart of me: why *do* I share? Upon reflection, I believe that sharing our authentic stories, particularly of struggle, of insecurity, of vulnerability, weaves a net of hands by which to catch others who may fall. Shared joys and revelations of meaning in medicine, motherhood, and the intersection of the two can help magnify our purpose and remind us of our blessings. It fuels understanding, empathy, and community. It requires trust, and it breeds trust. I hope in the pages to follow you will find some advice, some guiding principles, and some truth-telling that can support you and lift you up during your journey as a current or future mother in medicine.

Washington, DC, USA   Katherine Chretien, MD

Reference

1. Chretien KC. Paying at the pump. Ann Intern Med. 2008;148(8):622–3.

Acknowledgments

Were it not for the many women who have contributed to the Mothers in Medicine blog, this book would have never been. I am grateful to each one for pouring out a little of themselves onto the pages, sharing their laughter and struggles and everything in between. A special thank goes out to all of the "original cast" who embraced the idea of the blog and helped get it off to a running start including Terry, Liz, Artemis, Christie, Heather, Martina, Genevieve, Fizzy, Julia, Pathmom, Tatiana, Sarah, drwhoo, and Anesthesioboist. Terry, Heather, and Fizzy continue to be writers after 9 years earning them special MiM stripes for longevity: seeing you all blossom in your writing and careers and life over the years has been a treat. MiM stripes for prolificness go to Fizzy, Gizabeth, Monique, and Jalan. You have all contributed so importantly to the fabric of MiM with hundreds of posts combined. Gizabeth, thank you for your friendship and for being such a wonderful support to everyone.

The blog introduced me to Terry, who has become my academic collaborator, peer mentor, and friend. We now have offices close by in the Deans' Suite, something we couldn't have imagined during our first in-person meeting in the Children's National courtyard. Thank you for your encouragement, wise counsel, and support in this project and in all life/career projects.

To all the readers of MiM who sent in their questions, wrote guest posts, commented on posts, or just followed along, you are why we share. Thank you for being part of our community.

I am indebted to Janet Foltin, previously of Springer, who listened to my pitch at SGIM and who believed in this book from the very beginning. Thank you for not giving up on the idea and for your guidance. Margaret Burns, developmental editor, patiently shepherded the manuscript and all of its many authors. Miranda Finch of Springer took over this unconventional project and helped see it through. Thank you all for making this book a reality.

For all the chapter authors Terry, Ashley, Hilit, Raeshell, Monique, Andrea, Jenni, Fizzy, Miriam, Gizabeth, Dawn, Kat, Jane, Audrey, and Rebecca, thank you for being part of this project and contributing your voices. I am honored to call you my colleagues. Thank you also to Maria Latham for serving as a reader and helping as part of her medical school independent study project.

Finally, many thanks to my mother-in-law Jane, a chapter author, and my mother Jenny who are amazing examples of motherhood for me. And, always, thanks to my husband Jean-Paul and children Jolie, Jean-Luc, and Pascal who have made me the luckiest mother in medicine there is.

Contents

The original version of this book was revised. An erratum to this book can be found at
https://doi.org/10.1007/978-3-319-68028-6_12

Contributors

Dawn Baker, MD, MS University of Utah School of Medicine, Salt Lake City, UT, USA

Jane H. Chretien, MD, FACP Department of Internal Medicine, The George Washington University School of Medicine, Bethesda, MD, USA

Audrey P. Corson, MD, FACP Department of Internal Medicine, The George Washington University School of Medicine, Bethesda, MD, USA
Florida Atlantic University, Boca Raton, FL, USA

Andrea Flory, MD Washington, DC, USA

Terry Kind, MD, MPH Department of Pediatrics, Medical Education, Children's National/The George Washington University, Washington, DC, USA

Jenni Levy, MD, FAACH Jenni Levy, LLC, Allentown, PA, USA

Rebecca E. MacDonell-Yilmaz, MD, MPH Division of Pediatric Hematology/Oncology, Hasbro Children's Hospital, Providence, RI, USA

Freida McFadden, MD Mothers in Medicine, Washington, DC, USA

Hilit F. Mechaber, MD, FACP University of Miami Miller School of Medicine, Miami, FL, USA

Kathleen Y. Ogle, MD George Washington University School of Medicine and Health Sciences, Washington, DC, USA

Elizabeth Ann Seng, MD Baptist Health Medical Center, Little Rock, AR, USA

Miriam Stewart, MD Perelman School of Medicine at the University of Pennsylvania, Philadelphia, PA, USA

Raeshell Sweeting, MD Division of Surgical Oncology and Endocrine Surgery, Department of Surgery, Vanderbilt University, Nashville, TN, USA

Monique Tello, MD, MPH Massachusetts General Hospital/ Harvard Medical School, Boston, MA, USA

Ashley VanDercar, MD, JD Department of Psychiatry, Case Western Reserve University/University Hospitals, Cleveland, OH, USA

About the Authors

Dawn L. Baker (PracticeBalance) practices anesthesiology at the University of Utah School of Medicine. A former chemical engineer, she has traveled all over the world pursuing rock climbing, which led to a shift in her career path toward medicine to experience closer personal interactions with patients while using her knowledge in science. She is a writer, a blogger, a wannabe weight lifter and yoga practitioner, a wife, a cancer survivor, and a mom to one daughter and one whippet.

Jane H. Chretien is board certified in internal medicine and is a fellow of the ACP. She graduated from New Jersey College of Medicine and Harvard School of Public Health. Following residency at Bellevue/Cornell Medical Center and Memorial Sloan Kettering, she completed a fellowship in infectious diseases at Georgetown. After decades of employed status, she became a founding partner of Bethesda Physicians, PC. She is a MiM to two physician sons, one physician daughter-in-law, and grandmother to three beloved grandchildren.

Katherine Chretien (KC) is an assistant dean for student affairs and associate professor of medicine at the George Washington University School of Medicine and Health Sciences. She practices hospital medicine at the Washington, DC, VA Medical Center. Her passions include writing, medical education, and putting together a great outfit. She lives with her husband and three children in the Washington, DC, suburbs and enjoys spending her free time running slowly and cheering at her kids' soccer games. Katherine founded Mothers in Medicine in 2008, and it continues to be her labor of love.

Audrey P. Corson is board certified in internal medicine and is a fellow in the American College of Physicians. She graduated from the University of Colorado School of Medicine and did her residency at Duke and Mt. Zion/UCSF. In 2000, she cofounded Bethesda Physicians, PC, a practice consisting of four female internists. Since retiring in 2012, she has been on the faculty of the George Washington University School of Medicine and Health Sciences and Florida Atlantic University School of Medicine. She is currently the acting medical director of Mobile Med, a clinic for the uninsured and underinsured. She is a MiM to three children and three grandchildren.

Andrea Flory is a primary care internist and medical educator, most recently employed as creator and director of a course teaching clinical skills and reasoning to medical students. She is currently taking a short break from work as a Washington, DC, stay-at-home mom. Andrea is an ardent reader, cyclist, and inveterate creator of all sorts of things. She is enjoying the sojourn at home with her husband and 5-year-old son but looking forward to discovering her next career role.

Terry Kind (T) serves as the assistant dean for clinical education and is an associate professor of pediatrics at the George Washington University and Children's National. She has long enjoyed practicing primary care pediatrics at a community-based children's health center in an underserved region of Washington, DC. She is a mom, educator, pediatrician, researcher, and lifelong learner, and like many she experiences some overlap among those roles. Outside of the workday, she can be found doing a crossword puzzle, running uphill outside slowly, watching her daughter swim fast, or listening to her son and husband make music. She has been a long-time contributor to MiM since its inception and tweets @Kind4Kids.

Jenni Levy (Jay) is a third-generation physician who followed her father and both her grandfathers into medicine. She is an internist and hospice/palliative care physician. After 20 years in primary care practice and 10 years of hospice work, she is now a personal consultant providing guidance for advance planning and end-of-life care. Dr. Levy also teaches communication skills and relationship-centered care nationally through the American Academy on Communication in Healthcare. Her writing has appeared in the *New York Times*, the *Huffington Post*, *Pulse Magazine*, and the *Annals of Internal Medicine*. She lives in Allentown, PA, with her husband and daughter.

Rebecca E. MacDonell-Yilmaz (Beckster) is a pediatrician, wife, and mother of two little boys. She earned her BA and MPH from Dartmouth College and her MD from Stony Brook University School of Medicine. She completed her pediatrics residency and chief residency at Hasbro Children's Hospital in Providence, RI. She is currently completing fellowships in hospice and palliative medicine and pediatric hematology/oncology. She lives in RI and blogs about medicine and motherhood at The Growth Curve (www.thegrowthc.com).

Freida McFadden (Fizzy) is a mother of two and practicing physician specializing in physical medicine and rehabilitation. Her Kindle bestselling books have been featured on Student Doctor Network, AMWA, Medscape, KevinMD, Mothers in Medicine, and MedPage Today.

Hilit F. Mechaber is an associate dean for student services and associate professor of clinical medicine at the University of Miami Miller School of Medicine. In addition to practicing and teaching general internal medicine, she creates and oversees programs and resources for medical student support. Her professional niche is in the area of career development and work-life balance. Though she wishes she had more time to pursue her many hobbies, she is most passionate about her family. As the proud mom of two daughters, and married to a fellow academic general internist and dean of medical education, she can be spotted running 5Ks with the family, baking for others, cheering on the Miami Hurricanes, listening to Broadway musicals, and most of all enjoying her secret love of karaoke.

Kathleen Y. Ogle is an assistant professor at the George Washington University School of Medicine and Health Sciences. She blends her craft of emergency medicine with her educational hat in both the George Washington University Hospital and Washington, DC, VA Medical Center, molding medical minds to apply hands-on ultrasound, triage and treat in the ER, and develop as clinician educators. Her greatest love is her son, with whom she explores parks and trails, residing in Northern Virginia.

Elizabeth Ann Seng (Gizabeth Shyder) is a pathologist at Baptist Health Medical Center in Little Rock, AR. She is happily remarried to Stephan Seng, and they are co-raising Cecelia and Jack with the kid's dad and stepmom in addition to two precocious cats named Pink and Katybell. Gizabeth is a voracious reader and enjoys coffee, hiking, yoga, travel, music, and red wine (not necessarily in that order). She feels lucky to have intense passion for motherhood and pathology and to be able to do both.

Miriam Stewart (m) is a pediatrician, writer, and mindfulness practitioner. She is an assistant professor of clinical pediatrics at the Perelman School of Medicine at the University of Pennsylvania and a hospitalist at the Children's Hospital of Philadelphia where she also leads the Residency Wellness Program and cochairs the Program for Humanistic Medicine and Physician Wellbeing and the Narrative Medicine Program. She lives with her partner and daughter in Philadelphia.

Raeshell Sweeting (Cutter) is an assistant professor of surgery at Vanderbilt University where she focuses on breast cancer care. She is the associate program director of the Breast Surgical Oncology fellowship in addition to serving as a core faculty member on the Surgical Education Committee. She lives in Nashville with her spunky daughter and husband. In addition to hanging out with her family, she enjoys writing and making jewelry in her free time.

Monique Tello (Genmedmom) is an internist at MGH in Boston. Her clinical interests include diet, lifestyle, and work-life balance. She writes at her own blog Generallymedicine.com, is a regular contributor at Harvard Health Blog and Mothers in Medicine, and has written for NEJM Knowledge+ and KevinMD. She is married to local sports broadcaster Bob Socci, and they have two children.

Ashley VanDercar is a psychiatry resident at University Hospitals/Case Western. Prior to starting medical school, she practiced as an attorney and health-care risk manager. Before having a child, Ashley's pastimes included scuba diving, skydiving, and horseback riding. Since the birth of her son David, her free time has been occupied by more glorious pastimes, like building Lego castles and marathon-reading *Captain Underpants*.

Chapter 1
Choosing Motherhood and Medicine: The First Questions

Terry Kind

I'm in a little bit of a predicament, hoping you can help me. I'm a college junior, hoping to apply to medical school soon, but kind of at a difficult crossroads.

Let me preface this by saying that I'm 20 years old and I know that it's maybe too soon to start thinking about children. But, if there's one thing I know, it's that I was born to be a mom. I'll never admit that out loud to my college friends, but it's true. I've always loved children, and I've always felt that my future kids will have to be my number one priority in my life. However, my mom gave up her dreams to stay at home with my brother and I, and the regret and resentment she feels has really affected our family. I therefore try to over-compensate and promise myself I'll never radiate that kind of resentment towards my family in the future. But then I think, what if it's the other way around and I start to regret not having spent enough time with them? I consistently find myself up at 4 a.m. on your blog searching keywords like "balance", "regret"...you know, really healthy things to be thinking about at 4 a.m. ...

I know it's all kind of presumptuous and maybe silly that I haven't even stepped foot into a medical school yet (to look around or even interview for that matter), and I'm already worried about these things. But the thing is, medical school is an expensive road to go down, without being 100% in it. I keep reading these terrible horror stories about people who go into medicine and drop out during their third year after having used so many student loans, etc. And for goodness sakes, it seems like every other day some media outlet is coming out with a poll about how 50% or ___% of doctors wouldn't choose the road again if they could.

Gosh, it's all so confusing to me. I find myself taking screen-shots of the success stories, or "satisfied" or "happy" mom/doctor submissions on your blog, and printing it out to paste my "study" wall to help me trudge through this MCAT preparation, in attempts to keep me focused and dedicated. Can anyone out there give me insight or share some advice?

—Anonymous, "MiM Mail: Overthinking medicine as a career?" January 9, 2014

T. Kind, MD, MPH (✉)
Department of Pediatrics, Medical Education, Children's National/The George Washington University, 111 Michigan Ave NW, Washington, DC 20010, USA
e-mail: tkind@childrensnational.org

If you were to ask my children, they'd tell you their mother is qualified to write this chapter because she looks after their well-being and safety, only *sometimes* at the expense of fun. They appreciate the tragedies avoided and the extra knowledge they gain as a result of all the medical terminology. Yes, I am a mother of a teen girl who is an avid reader, fast butterfly swimmer, strong in self-esteem and intellect, and at times a stellar big sister to her tween brother. He too is keenly intelligent, and he will make music with anything and everything. And when I am working in the land of academia, I am engrossed in curricular planning, teaching, research, and also providing pediatric primary care to children in a community-based inner-city health center. And none of this would be feasible nor meaningful without the support and patience of the love of my life; how lucky I am to have him as my partner.

In this chapter you'll find the questions we mothers in medicine ask ourselves and the questions we hear from others starting out on this journey. First off, let's consider which came first, being a mother or being in medicine. Then let's address questions about who we are, what we do, and what we've chosen. The chapter concludes with the ten best things about being a mother in medicine, and yes it was hard to limit myself to just ten. And finally, some practical tips and things to reflect on further as you navigate this book, our blog, and your journey.

Which Came First, Being a Mother or Being in Medicine?

This answer will vary, and that's okay. There is no right answer; only the answer that is right for any given individual in the context of her family and goals. Moreover, one could instead ask which came first, the *idea* to become a mother or the idea to go into medicine? For me, the idea that I would be a mother someday came way back when, as a kid, I imagined college, falling in love, and making babies, in that order. But there wasn't much thought to the rest at that point. As a child in junior high, I didn't know that school (training, continuing education, additional degrees, academia) can be nearly a lifelong endeavor. Both of my non-physician nonmedical parents had gone to graduate school. I forgot to worry or wonder about how the additional years of school and the rest of one's professional career factors in to family.

Fall in love I did, but I also fell for the marvels of the human body, health promotion, disease prevention, and treatment planning. And hence came the next steps in my schooling. I established my career before motherhood. But in the back of my mind, I knew at some point there'd be a family. And there it was in the back—not the forefront—of my mind.

Until it was in the forefront of my mind. Eventually, as my nonmedical friends with whom I had graduated from college were having their babies, or trying to do so with varying degrees of success, I began to feel some urgency. Urgency, because like many a diligent medical school graduate who feels she has the very conditions she is studying, I somehow "knew" it would take me years of trying before I would see two lines appear on the beta HCG stick. And yet in reality, pregnancy came easily, and I joined the motherhood club, twice. Having moved beyond the questions of *whether* motherhood and medicine would happen, it was time to address the questions of *how* it would work out.

Questions We Hear

Students and others early in their training ask mothers in medicine some common questions, such as, "Should I go into medicine if I know I want to be a mother?" And then there are others who ask, "I'm a mother, should I go into medicine?" All askers want to know, can it be done, and can it (both) be done well?

And the answer is…

There are several right answers. One is, *yes*! Another answer is, *try it and see*! Still another approach to answering that question is that you can do both well, but you will be better at one or the other at various times throughout your life, throughout your kids' lives, and throughout your career.

Finally, another reasonable response is to ask a different question instead. Rather than asking, *should I go into medicine if I know I want children (or already have children)*, instead ask, *what career will I enjoy enough so that my time spent at work away from my children feels rewarding*. I look back on the beginning of parenting and know that I could never have gone back to work after parental leave (twice) to a job that I did not like. So ask, will that job be a career in medicine? Will I be able to give of myself in service to my patients, and in educating a range of trainees, *and* be able to start and end each day ready for the ups and downs of love and family and caregiving?

Do also ask yourself what will rejuvenate you at the end of a long day (or long night) at work. And then *do* those things. Rejuvenation will likely come through sleep, good food, exercise plus a hobby or two, plus spending time with your family. These days, for me, that family time is in part spent chauffeuring to and from swim team, music lessons, karate, their friends' houses, more music, and more swimming. Ever an optimist, I see those very rides as an opportunity for togetherness, depending on their readiness to chat… sometimes, somewhat surprisingly, more is shared on some topics (think: puberty) when both conversational partners are facing forward in the car.

The "me time" that I take to refresh outside of pure work or pure parenting includes multiple attempts at the Sunday *New York Times* crossword puzzle and getting out for a jog a few times per week. Small pleasures lead to large gains in wellness.

That Other Question We Physicians Get, Particularly in Pediatrics

Even before I was personally thinking about having children, well before I *had* children, back when serving as seasoned resident and as a new attending, my focus was nonetheless on children and families because after all, I am a pediatrician. And when periodically asked by the parents of my patients, "Do you have kids?" I knew that question could mean one of two things. It was either pointed at my apparent inexperience or more benevolently at my seeming like I *must* have children because of my adept pediatric display of skills with their children. Fortunately for me (and for my patients), it was more often the latter. But it did make me think about the following common questions we hear.

Did Being a Doctor Make You a Better Mother or Being a Mother Make You a Better Doctor? Are You a Better Physician **Because** *You Have Kids?*

> *I never went into medicine to become a better mother. I never became a mother to become a better doctor. But, the two journeys merged in 2013 when I knew something was seriously wrong with my almost six year-old son... The mother inside of me was strong during the five days [in the hospital], and the doctor inside of me was quick to decline any unnecessary blood draws and made sure that he got out that hospital as quickly as possible.*
>
> —Anonymous, "Guest post: Trust me, I am mother," February 4, 2015

> *Motherhood has given me a more zen-like patience with which to approach the craziness and chaos of medicine and residency.... I can't do it all and I know it. However I will still try... I love sharing my life with my daughter, therefore while at work I am even more motivated to make it count for something, to 'help people' as she tells me, to heal, to learn, to affect change. She has inspired my medicine in ways that make every struggle of motherhood well worth the gain in every aspect of who I am.*
>
> —Cutter, "How motherhood changed my medicine," December 28, 2013

> *Medicine has taught me how to be strong for other people.*
>
> —m, "For the better and for the worse but mostly for the better," December 13, 2013.

As a pediatrician, I am asked this quite often. By students, by residents, by patients, by patients' families, by trainees, by colleagues, by neighbors, and so on. I try to answer sincerely, but because I resist the notion that one is not as good at being a pediatrician if he or she does not have kids, I don't want to fall back on the easy answer that I'm better at it now that I have two darlings myself. Even with all the overlap that parenting as a pediatrician entails, having experienced breastfeeding and children with nursemaid's elbow (also known as radial head subluxation, and multiple times at that), sleep associations, one febrile UTI, the barking cough and stridor of croup, and now acne, puberty, and more.

However, because I want to rush home promptly—if not early—from work to be with my kids and arrive late to work periodically when I practically never did so before motherhood, maybe (for these and other reasons) I'm a worse physician. But not really. With more to do, more to care about, and no more hours in the day, efficiency is essential. And yet, efficiency isn't everything.

Mothers in medicine like me, will ask themselves, can I do both, and can I do both well? We fear we will do one well and the other poorly, or possibly do both poorly. Truth is, over time and with experience we become better at both, but not always along the same slope, and it is not a steady trajectory of improvement. That is, there are plenty of parenting problems and job-related challenges along the way. Like when your office adds on Saturday hours when it was previously a Monday through Friday gig, or when there's that school field trip that you thought your child wouldn't care if you arranged to come or not, but then he mentions last minute that he wants you to come along. The ultimate goal? To be what you love to be and do what you love to do. And, when you are with the ones you love, and when you are doing what you love to do, aim to really be there. Do both parenting and the profession proudly, be a mother in medicine who works toward mastery but knows that mistakes are not failures. It's what you do with the mistakes. It's how you grow and help others grow.

Questions of Identity

Once You're a Mother, Are You Ever Not a Mother?

And it is a long road to medicine, so once you are in medicine, you *typically* remain in medicine, but that is not a given. You can take a break from blogging about motherhood, and perhaps there is time on some evenings when you don't open your laptop, or some weekends when you aren't seeing patients or responding to emails, and you can take a break from being a doctor (neighbors' and friends' and family members' medical questions and text messages notwithstanding). But the *being* the mother and the *being* in medicine is pretty much all the time, even when it's not fully there. The motherhood is mostly always there, because even if at the "most important" work meeting or during patient care visits or a scholarly conference, you know you are on call for everything parent-related, such as that time the school bus didn't come, the monkey bars were slippery, they can't find those new pencils you bought, or other minor and major emergencies, or just when your kids want to chat, smart phones are ever-present.

But are there times when you aren't a mother? Or aren't in medicine? Do you turn off one while doing the other? Is that possible? Or are the two aspects of your identity intertwined? How does it feel to be both at all times? The *mother* portion of me as a mother in medicine feels particularly bad leaving my family to head in to work on a snow day. The *medicine* portion of me as a mother in medicine feels good, to be in a service profession, indeed. And when my children happen to notice that my job entails service to others, and they are proud of that, well that's another positive thing about being both. And then, as for *doing* both, think about how you answer the following.

What Do You Do?

My mother, not in medicine, and this mother in medicine, went to have a biopsy. Her biopsy. By a surgeon. I am not a surgeon. Nor am I a doctor for adults. My day to day is infants, toddlers, school-aged children, tweens, and adolescents. And medical students.

How does your mom introduce you to her doctors? My mother introduced me to the surgeon whom she herself was just meeting at that moment, as her daughter. Sounds reasonable. Started off well. Though this was immediately followed by, "She's a pediatrician." I paused briefly at the stark declaration, and softly came up with, "...who knows nothing about what you do."

Why did I demur? Why so modest? The surgeon and I might indeed speak the same language (though she much more tersely). But I need not hover, make her nervous, nor imply that the reason I'm there is because I'm a doctor too. The reason I was there was to support my mother. As a daughter.

But alas, I guess I was also there because I do speak, or at least understand, that language.

—T, "Being introduced," February 10, 2013

How do you introduce yourself, at work, with patients, at parties, at your kids' elementary school, to the new neighbors? There was that time when I was shoe shopping and was mistaken for a waitress because of the comfortable clogs I sought. You know the ones. And I didn't correct them. Another hardworking service profession. But different.

Some mothers in medicine describe purposefully not outing themselves as physicians, at trips to the doctor with their kids or their own parents, at the playground, on the plane with your own crying child, at girl scout meetings. Quaintly, I had to show my BLS-CPR certification card to be a first aider for my child's extracurricular camping activity. Fortunately, it was up to date. And hence I could inspect and then remove the tick (or was it a splinter), administer the albuterol, place an Ace wrap, ensure that everyone brushes their teeth even when sleeping in a tent, *and* that all seat belts are fastened en route. Mothering, and in medicine.

What Does It Mean to Choose Motherhood and Medicine?

Choice has played a significant role in women's lives whether over our bodies or our names or what's for dinner. And here, the choice to be both a mother and in medicine. Two hugely fulfilling, all consuming, give it your all, foster the growth, health, and well-being of others, most rewarding of positions. While still being who we are—as individuals—beyond our motherhood and our medical roles.

I chose my husband, but didn't know how we would grow together to find the best balance of parenting and pediatrics, together. Choosing implies doing something deliberately, but choice also means variety. You can choose how you want to parent, but you can't choose your children's personalities. You *can* work on choosing a new job, but can't choose new kids.

Fortunately, my kids feel proud of my choices, and periodically let that be known, sometimes in the subtle ways they talk to their friends.

What do my kids think about having a mother who chose medicine (and in their case, a father as well)? On the whole they are proud, and they periodically express this, among other things, over the years:

There was that time while out to dinner as a family on a Saturday evening when we ran into my colleague at a restaurant, and I couldn't help but mention that I had been at work all day. And my son said, "But mom, for you, work is fun, so it's not so bad that you had to work on Saturday." Moreover, I was inspired when my children came to their own realization that it is okay if I need to go in to work on the occasional weekend day, because they want those in need to have a doctor available.

My children were happy to serve as history and physical diagnosis examples for the local medical school's pediatric student interest group. Free cardiology, orthopedic, and ear, nose, and throat exams. Normal variants on display.

Children of mothers in medicine know how to get us to let them stay up later, with a mere, clever ask. Does this bedtime routine sound familiar? Like many children, ours want to stay up just a little bit later. And they are so very in tune to what will motivate the physician parent. And in turn what will allow them a few more minutes (hours??) of wakeful banter. When they want to stay up even later than their working parents already let them, all they need to ask is just one little question that goes something like this, "Mommy, can you tell me again how the heart pumps the blood around the body?" Or perhaps, "Will you remind me how the lungs work again?" It can happen whether we are pulmonologists or cardiologists or in primary care or even a health services researcher might succumb to an innocent query such as, "Can you review regression analysis for the social determinants of health just one more time?" We are weak when it comes to an opportunity to explain what we love to do, that is, what we do at work as our primary involvement when we are not with our precious little ones. And they know with that simple question, "How does the food get all the way from my mouth to my large intestine?" (or even more enticing, to ask where the food goes after that) and they have bought themselves more not-yet-sleeping mother-in-medicine time.

And there's the not-so-subtle pride, as I overhear, daughter to a friend, "Oh, did you hurt yourself because my mother is a doctor so she can help you." And the friend responds, "I know you've told me that a million times."

For this chapter I asked my own children what they liked about having a medical mom (in our case, both parents). They told me that they love that everyone in the neighborhood (read: their friends' parents) come to us with medical questions. And they like that they don't have to travel to go to the doctor. They also liked that when we do take them to the doctor, we "know everyone" and "everything" so it's just like getting together with friends. And finally, they said that they feel glad that they get to stay healthy. If only we had that built in mother-in-medicine insurance!

One commenter on MiM (an 18-year-old daughter of a physician) shared this:

> On behalf of children everywhere with doctor parents who worry, fret, and guilt themselves over the time they have to spend apart from their children...I want you to know that we love you, and even if it's hard when we're little to understand what you do, or why you're gone so long sometimes (though we tend to vaguely grasp even then the idea that "work" is very hard and busy and keeps you away even though you love us very much and wish all the time that you were here with us), we're proud of you and love you very much. We do our best to understand and accept these struggles with you, and we see better while looking back from older ages all of the sacrifices and difficulties you've endured for us, and just how much you've always loved us--and at all ages young to old, we love to hear you say it on nights when you're around to tuck us into bed.
>
> —Anonymous, "Guest post: A comment from a daughter," July 8, 2008

What Are the Ten Best Things About Being a Mother in Medicine?

1. Fewer trips to the doctor.
2. We have special skills, as in the bandages we apply are just perfect.
3. With all that we see and do at work, we don't have to sweat the small stuff at home.
4. It just keeps getting better. Every age is an interesting age, an age to marvel at the growth and/or change. As can be the case for our career as well.
5. To vaccinate? Easy (science-based, preventive health) decision.
6. Literarily, good medicine is a metaphor for motherhood and vice versa, particularly when it comes to facilitating health, caregiving, and caring.
7. Additional opportunities for the placebo effect.
8. Physicians are caregivers. We care about kids and families.

9. Bonding with other mothers and other mothers in medicine, taking comfort in the similarities and the differences in ourselves, our kids, our paths, but knowing that there is such a range of what's "right" and different definitions of successes.
10. Our kids make us better humans, and that makes us better at what we do every day.

Practical Tips and Things to Reflect On

- There is no one "right" time to have a family. It will work out if you are able to enlist support from others, and keep a balance, and reshuffle priorities as things change over time.
- It may in fact take a village. Have or grow a support system (your extended family and friends) accessible to you.
- Being a parent and being a physician can both be all encompassing. It's okay to ask for help.
- Plan and organize, but be ready to throw out those plans when necessary.
- Be present where you are. If you are with your children, *be with* your children.
- On the other hand, know how to multitask!
- Use your commute not just to get from one place to the other but to transition from motherhood to medicine or vice versa. Plus, books on tape, music, and podcasts!
- Weigh all the things that are important to you that give you meaning and fulfillment, but be ready to have those things change over time and be open to re-prioritizing.
- Find sources of renewal. Your kids themselves. Your significant others. Alone time. Since your goal is to do two things, motherhood and medicine, allow one to help you reclaim the joy in the other.

Chapter 2
Having and Raising Children During Physician Training: Medical School

Ashley VanDercar and Hilit F. Mechaber

> I'm a med student with a baby. I get asked all the time how I 'do' it. Some weeks, it's no big deal, it's not that bad, and I feel the balance works well for our little family. But when she brings me her favorite book to read, pulls the charger out of the computer, and screams until I read to her, I think to myself that I don't know if I can 'do' this, or even if I want to.
>
> I have friends who have babies, too. One is a full time SAHM. Her instagram pictures of nature walks, arts and crafts, and 'Sunday/Monday/EVERYDAY Funday' kill me a little bit inside. Another friend works from home and her pictures of 'lunch with the little prince!' make me sigh/roll my eyes/shake my head (depending on the day, the most recent Histology quiz, or whether I got to see my baby before heading out in the morning).
>
> I picked priorities. She was drinking formula at 3 months (end of summer vacation) but I made all my own baby food. Her grandma takes her to music class once a week since I can't, but I put her to sleep every night. We read books and play all day Saturday, but Sunday mornings I go out to study.
>
> My husband is awesome and supportive and doesn't understand how I can love the field of medicine, love school (nerd, I know) and still feel so conflicted. I guess that's the imperfect side of living your dream- other dreams sometimes get put to the side for a bit.
>
> But as imperfect as the balancing act seems, when my baby is teething and only wants her mommy- and, since it is 3am, I am home (and awake), or when I get that HUGE smile and kiss when I come home, it feels so perfect. I'm sure some researcher somewhere has proven that listing bones, ligaments, and muscle attachments as a bedtime story, and speaking in mnemonics for disease presentations helps kids go really far in life. And keeps them happy. Here's to hoping.
>
> —Boxes, "Guest post: When Imperfect feels like Perfect," May 2, 2013

A. VanDercar, MD, JD
Department of Psychiatry, Case Western Reserve University/University Hospitals,
10524 Euclid Ave, Walker Building, 8th Fl, Cleveland, OH 44106, USA
e-mail: ashley.vandercar@uhhospitals.org

H.F. Mechaber, MD, FACH (✉)
University of Miami Miller School of Medicine,
1611 NW 10th Ave, Suite 2155, Miami, FL 33136, USA
e-mail: hmechabe@med.miami.edu

© Springer International Publishing AG 2018
K. Chretien (ed.), *Mothers in Medicine*,
https://doi.org/10.1007/978-3-319-68028-6_2

Hilit Mechaber

You did it! You were accepted to medical school, and, professionally, you are on the road to realizing your dream of becoming a physician. But like many women before you, you're planning your future, your *entire* future, and how you will possibly have time to be the best doctor, partner, and mother, all at the same time. Those of us who are parents now, and reflect back on how we managed to have and raise our children, know that we all asked the famous question: "When is the best time to have children during medical training?" As you will likely learn, there is no one size fits all answer. For many, even the best attempt at making perfect plans can be met with a variety of outcomes. While some women are lucky to have biology on their side and hopefully to their advantage, many others can share stories of the trials and tribulations, frustrations, and downright surprises that come along with the hopes and dreams of motherhood.

There is so much to consider when having and raising children during medical school, that the thought alone can be overwhelming. Some will come to medical school having already experienced the joys and challenges of motherhood but are about to see some of those stressors explode exponentially. As a student affairs dean for over 9 years and medical student mentor and advisor for almost two decades, I have advised and supported many medical students who have successfully managed to have children during medical school. In this chapter, one of my former students Ashley shares her incredible story about managing all 4 years of medical school as a single parent by choice. Others, though, will want to hold onto the hopes of having control in planning for their futures. Why not? We are so used to meticulously crafting every next step of our personal and professional lives, so planning for children should not be any different. If planning is an option and in your favor, then timing of children in medical school can potentially make a big difference. Yet each woman is an individual, and factors important to one may be less important to others. Give yourself time to think, plan ahead, and communicate with those who will be part of your support system. Identify that support network, and if you are lacking one, reach out to those in your medical school administration who can guide and direct you to resources that may be of help. As you'll read in Ashley's account, creativity was key, and asking for help was part of her strategy for success.

Timing

Premedical School Questions and Choices

If you will have the chance to plan for the birth of your child, there are important aspects you can review, possibly even influencing your choice of medical schools. If you anticipate having children while you are in medical school, you will want to review the curriculum, grading policies, student support systems, and campus resources, including healthcare, health insurance, and even childcare on campus. In many healthcare systems where medical schools are located, resources may differ for faculty, staff, and students. Some medical schools are located within a healthcare system, others are connected to parent universities, and therefore access to resources differs. So reach out to the deans and administrative officers who can provide you with accurate information as you make important decisions for you and your future family. It's also best not to surprise anyone with the exciting news of your pregnancy. There is a lot that your administration will want to help you plan, and keeping things a secret might be more of a hindrance than you know. Things you may not think about, like your time in the gross anatomy lab and potential exposure to formaldehyde, for example, will be important for others to explain and guide you. The more you plan and communicate, the better off you'll be. Explore your options earlier than later so you remain informed along the way and can make the best choices for you and your baby.

Preclinical vs. Clinical Years

Invest in exploring your curriculum and the differences in responsibilities between your preclinical and clinical years. One of the major differences between having a child before or during your clinical clerkships is the amount of flexibility in the curriculum and schedule. Remember that pregnancy is not a disability, and as such, any medical issues you face during pregnancy or after your delivery would be managed by your school in the same way as any other medical issues. Most medical schools teach the preclinical curriculum in a sequential manner, with each new class building on the foundation of the prior one. So as you move along through your first 18–24 months of your curriculum, if you needed to take a substantial amount of time off, you'll need to be familiar with your school's policies around a leave of absence. While the administration will grant you the time you desire or may need medically, this time off during year 1 or 2 might ultimately translate into an entire year off. This is not something that everyone plans for and also has important financial implications, so it is important to ask and understand. As a preclinical student, how many hours per week are you usually expected to be in class? Are you at a school where class attendance is not always required, and are there options for remote learning? Personal questions to consider: Will you have time and a quiet location to study? Can you dedicate a substantial amount of time to your studies, and will you have some help managing childcare needs at times of increased stress on you as a student (i.e., pre-exams and during your preparation for national board exams)?

Students who have their first children during medical school often feel that the clinical years are more forgiving, only in terms of scheduling. Traditionally, the core junior clerkships run between 4, 6, and 8 weeks, with natural breaks in between. Some curricula have longitudinal experiences where this may not apply. But for the most part, students find that having a baby in year 3 or 4 can lend itself to a natural "break." Often students will choose this option when possible and work with their schools to also take extended time off either during the end of pregnancy or at the time of delivery. While not a formal "maternity leave," because students are not employees, similar time is given as needed, without any academic penalty. Things to consider again have to do with finances and also desires to graduate on time. Each student will have to consider this individually, but many find that taking extended time off gives them flexibility to enjoy the first few months of motherhood with less stress of the clinical clerkship years. If your medical school allows for some flexibility in scheduling between your third and fourth year, then options to spread out the curricular requirements may also allow you some more time to devote to board exams, residency interviews, and preparing for that transition later on.

So, if planning is your strength, and the stars align and give you some control over this important life decision, then there is *a lot* you can think about and should think about ahead of time. But sometimes, no matter how much planning you do, you realize that you will learn best under fire. Ashley's stories of her struggles and successes highlight just how amazing, strong, and resourceful we women can be and that you too can make motherhood work during medical school. Buckle up for the ride!

Ashley VanDercar

Two months after my emergent cesarean section, I was lying in bed trying to catch some much needed sleep when the phone rang. I received fairly unexpected news: I had been accepted off the waitlist into the University of Miami Medical School. At first I was overjoyed. Then the reality of the situation sank in. I would be leaving all of my family in Tampa to go to Miami—just me and my infant son. You see: I am a single mom. A single mom by choice. My darling baby boy was made with the help of a reproductive endocrinologist and a carefully selected sperm donor.

Fast-forward a little over 4 years: somehow, I survived medical school. Everyday was a struggle, but I made it. Perhaps because of that experience I am now exceptionally happy. I am working 60+ h a week as a psychiatry resident, but due to the tricks I learned during those 4 years, I am able to maintain a great work-life balance.

How to survive being a medical student + a mother:

- Be superwoman.
- I'm not joking. Be superwoman: overly *organized and efficient.*
- Let go of some of your pride: *ask for help.*
- *Accept imperfection* and don't feel guilty about it.
- *Expect a lot* from your child, they will surprise you.

Organization and Efficiency

Every morning, when I dropped my son off at day-care, the staff would chide me to "slow down." But slowing down was not an option. There was too much to do. As long as I kept going, pedal-to-the-metal, I could slow down at home in the morning and evening. Those special times of the day were my own version of family time.

As a mom in medical school, you have to throw your idea of parenthood out the window. You develop your own style. When you are working 6 days a week on a surgery rotation, getting home at 8 PM only to wake up at 4 AM, you must have your priorities straight: remaining sane. You do not want to stumble out of bed, make breakfast, pack a lunch, get your child into his clothes, serve breakfast, and then find yourself screaming at your child to hurry up because you are inevitably running late.

Before he learned to dress himself, I often put my son to bed wearing his clothes for the next day. As he got older, I began laying piles of clothes out for the entire week. He could choose his outfit and get himself dressed. This worked so well I started doing the same thing for myself. The pile included every accouterment, including underwear and socks. This cuts down on the inevitable last-minute search for matching socks.

To avoid a hurried breakfast, I made a mini-Crock-Pot each night before going to bed. I also set the breakfast table. Sometimes I made steel-cut oats, sometimes a French-toast casserole. It varied. Either way, I had a hot breakfast ready to go when I rolled out of bed.

I did not wake my son up until I was done getting ready. We were then able to have quality time during a leisurely breakfast.

School lunches took a while to figure out. The trick I eventually learned was to buy bento boxes and spend 30 min each Sunday making a week's lunches. Every month I froze up a bunch of mini-pizzas and PBJ sandwiches in vacuum-sealed bags. I made dinner in the Crock-Pot twice a week and froze several servings for especially hectic evenings.

Tips for Organization and Efficiency

- Develop your own routine—you are not a normal parent.
- Be highly efficient so you don't have to be hurried at home.
- As you fold laundry, immediately put it into "outfit" piles, for both yourself and your child.
- Invest in two good Crock-Pots: a small one for breakfasts and a big one (with a timer) for dinners.
- Make and pack school lunches ahead of time—get five high-quality bento boxes and fill them up on Sunday.

Ask for Help

I've always had difficulty accepting help from others. But, being a parent in medical school makes you realize that there are certain things in life you just cannot do alone.

There's this nifty little sticker that schools send home that says: "picture day is tomorrow." All of the other kids in my son's class had their sticker placed on their take-home folder. My child came home wearing his sticker smack-dab in the middle of his back. His teachers realized it was the only way to ensure I remembered picture day.

One of the biggest challenges of being a mother in medical school was childcare. Medical students and residents have very unpredictable schedules. It is hard enough to find affordable childcare that is available beyond the typical 8–5 PM schedule. When you add a lack of predictability, things become nearly impossible. In fact, one evening, I had a mandatory session on how to perform a pap smear (with a standardized patient). I couldn't find childcare! I ended up bringing my then 2-year-old son along—one of the nurses watched him out in the hallway. He sat there the entire hour, watching Netflix.

The most difficult period begins in the third year of medical school, when clinical rotations begin. Logistically, things get tricky. You often have to pre-round as early as 5:30 AM and then stay for admissions until 5 PM. But, 5 PM doesn't really mean 5 PM. It means that if someone comes in at 4:49 PM, you are there until much later. Similarly, during surgery rotations, cases scheduled to be 2 hours long often take at least twice that.

This was very problematic. When I learned how unpredictable my schedule would be (a few months before third year started), I sat down with my student services dean. We even started talking about whether I could go to school "part-time," only to realize that wouldn't solve the underlying problem. So, I became hell-bent on finding a solution.

I started my quest by making a flyer. I put my son's picture on it, a blurb with "my story," and the details of what I was looking for. I posted it all over his day-care, my condo building, and the medical school. Then I made an online version of the flyer and posted it on the medical school Facebook page. This paid off.

I found a delightful young couple—both first-year medical students—who were willing to wake up as early as 5 AM to watch my son and then drive him to school. I also found a teacher's aide at his school, with two children of her own, who took my son home with her at night when I couldn't get out in time. During interview season, she kept him for days on end.

This was pricey—but much cheaper than hiring a nanny. Plus, a little known fact is that the financial aid office can increase your loan amount to cover childcare costs. That was a huge help.

Tips for Managing Childcare Responsibilities During Medical School

- Attack the childcare dilemma full force and use all of your available resources, including social media.
- Make sure people know that you are in a tough situation and that you need all the help they can give you.
- Tell your colleagues about any time restraints you have.

Juggling life and parenting responsibilities particularly during the clinical years is likely the hardest part of having children during medical school. Schedules are unpredictable, you lack sleep, and you need to learn to take care of other people (your patients) while taking care of yourself and your children and/or family. Support, in any way you define it, will be the most important part of your success. Not all are fortunate enough to have family or a partner with whom to share these responsibilities. If that is indeed an option, then this may be a good reason why students choose to have their children born during their medical school years. If there is no set support to count on, reach out to anyone you can to help establish those networks so you can be as focused as possible at the times you do need to be at work.

Accept Imperfection! Redefine Your Successes

Some people might judge me for leaving my son with such a variety of caregivers. I questioned myself at times. It was the only way to survive medical school. I've now discovered that these experiences helped him become an amazing kid. He can sleep anywhere, can be moved from place to place while sleeping, and doesn't bat an eye at being left in the care of a stranger. In fact, he has an uncanny ability to charm people into doing his bidding.

Another difficulty was trying to study on the weekends. The weekend before my first final, I hired a nanny to watch my then 6-month-old son. That allowed me to study. But it cost well over a hundred dollars. It was not sustainable.

Next, I tried setting up a playpen with tons of toys, so I could study. That did not work. Eventually I bought a fisher-price iPad case, downloaded Netflix, and set my son up with "educational" cartoons. I felt horrible! But, I couldn't think of any other option. He is now 4 years old, and I promise those innumerable hours of watching PBS did not scar him for life. Shortly before preschool, I bought him an alphabet book and was shocked to learn that he had learned his entire alphabet from "Super Why" (a cartoon).

When you are working obscene hours, only to come home and have to study, you cannot fuss about being the perfect mom. You have to do what works for you and your family. It is more important that you feel sane—and not turn into a fire-breathing monster—than that you fulfill the demands put upon the typical mother.

Tips for Accepting Imperfection

- Do not look to others for validation—do what works for you, even if it runs contrary to what others consider "normal."
- Realize that you are not going to break your kid by letting him or her binge on PBS kids or other kid-friendly shows.

Most mothers in medicine are well aware of the adage, "you can have it all, just not all at the same time." Motherhood in medical training and especially in medical school will test your limits and your strength. It is critical that you define your own personal priorities and recognize that there is only one you, and you can only be the best that you can be on any given day. You are used to comparing yourselves to others, and most likely, you've been at the top of that competitive curve for a very long time, or you would not be in medical school! But now you are balancing so much more than only you, and each day the balance may tip a little. Try not to be your own worst enemy, and go easy on yourself. Allow yourself to define your successes perhaps in ways that you are not accustomed to. Lean on others, family, partners, or friends, and speak up when things are not going well. There will be days and times when you feel that you could have done things better, tried harder, worked more, scored higher, etc. When those little eyes look your way and smiles are directed at YOU, no matter how little you managed to study that day or whether you gave a perfect presentation or not does not matter to the little person who is looking at you. Your child thinks you're perfect and that needs to be your most important thought for the day!

Expect a Lot From Your Child

I'm warm and fuzzy and have a great relationship with my son. But I also expect a lot and tolerate nothing less. When my son was a toddler, I let him "cry it out" at bedtime. Initially he cried for over an hour. I was in tears myself. But this approach worked. He can now go to sleep in any setting, simply by being told to "go to bed."

I couldn't spend my evenings battling with my child about going to bed. I had to study. I chose the controversial method of "cry it out." It worked great.

Similarly, I did not clean up after my child. He had to clean up on his own. From the age of 2 to 4, the rule was fairly straightforward—he could not get a new toy out until the last one was put away. At the age of 4, I changed tactics, because it became more important to allow him "freedom" to play with many toys at once. Any toy left out after bedtime was taken away for 24 hours. We made it a game. We pretended there was a toy-eating monster in our house (we would then laugh about how silly that was) who only came out after bedtime. No matter how much of a mess there is, my son always cleans up all his toys at night. He does it with great glee. I only take away toys a few times a year.

Another thing that helps simplify life is that I expect him to eat whatever foods I eat. I refuse to be a short-order cook. I can't. I don't have the time. If he doesn't want what I'm serving, he can wait until the next meal to eat.

Please do not think my child goes hungry. He has developed an adult palate. He relishes Roquefort cheese and regularly tells people how his favorite two foods are broccoli and golden berries. Similarly, while meals are a leisurely affair, they are not playtime. If he gets up before a meal is done, the plate is taken away.

These types of expectations have allowed me to enjoy my time with my son. Other than vacations, we haven't had large chunks of time together. That was especially true during my third year of medical school. But, the time we have had together has been true quality time. I haven't constantly had to remind him to clean up his toys or stay at the table. I haven't had to scurry around the kitchen trying to make meals on demand. Instead, he has become a part of my life.

Tips for Expecting a Lot From Your Child

- Don't underestimate your child's ability to be a productive member of your family.
- Expect a lot from them, so that the time you do have together isn't monopolized by admonitions to behave.

The key thing to remember about having a child in medical school is that you are not a normal parent. Your child needs to become part of *your* life. Not the other way around. You already decided to become a doctor. That isn't going to change just because you have kids. Things will seem tough, and you will feel guilty. But remember: children are extremely resilient, and adapt to their circumstances. As long as you stay organized and efficient and enjoy your time together, you will survive. In fact, your child will probably flourish.

I have been tired since May 2015. I am so, so tired. But the sleep deprivation proved to be worth it today. You see, today was Match Day. The results were good. Outstanding, really. Not only did I match to my number one ranked program, but my future institution is one of the most prestigious medical centers in the world.

My journey to get to today was not easy. It took me three application cycles to get accepted into medical school. The emotional toll alone of receiving dozens of rejection letters is enough to make anyone go a little crazy. But with application cycles also comes time, and as we all know, with time comes a decline in ovarian function. Women physicians are all too familiar with that line graph comparing ovarian reserve to a woman's age. I was finally accepted into medical school at 27. By that time I was married to a man nine years my senior who was very eager to start a family. So we decided to have a baby… while I was in medical school.

(continued)

After a pregnancy complicated by complete placenta previa, studying for Step 1 in the height of my third trimester, and a major placental bleed during third year orientation- my beautiful Ben was born. I have loved my son with every ounce of my being since the second I heard him cry. He has brought our family indescribable joy and not a moment goes by that I am not thankful to have him.

But being a parent is even harder than I imagined (I still have PTSD from the newborn period). Being a parent while in medical school seems like an almost insurmountable challenge. It has been exhausting and challenging and there were times I did not think I would make it to today. But today is proof. When I celebrated the news of my match, I got to share that moment with my loving husband and our smart, wild, daring, and sweet little boy.

Yes, I am still exhausted. And no, I do not believe I will get to catch up on sleep anytime soon. But just as my increasing age correlates to my declining ovarian function (that damn graph), it also represents the passage of time. My grandmother used to say that the days were long but the years were short. So to all the women who wonder if they can be a mom while in medicine... the answer is YES. Do whatever is right for you and your individual circumstance. And if you do have a baby in medical school (or at any point in your medical career), there will be times when it's awful and times you genuinely don't believe you can do it anymore... but it is so worth it. And whatever you do, enjoy every second because my grandmother was right. There were so many long days, but these sweet, sweet years are ever so short.

—Maria Latham, "Guest post: Finally," March 24, 2017

Chapter 3
Having and Raising Children During Physician Training: Residency

Raeshell Sweeting

Guilt was one of the first feelings I experienced upon learning I was pregnant with my daughter, now 4 years old.

I had been on a pub crawl the night before, gotten home around 2 am and woke up a few hours later miserably sick. This might seem to be expected after a night out on the town, but I had gone to bed sober and hadn't drunk that much. I had taken a pregnancy test a few weeks earlier, prompted more by nausea and fatigue than a missed period as stress-induced amenorrhea was not new to me. It was negative.

That morning, not able to shake the fact there was something very wrong, I took a (second) pregnancy test. Positive. I took another. Positive. I took another. (still) Positive.

Pregnant, drinking, not taking folic acid, and ignoring what my body had been telling me for weeks, which was have some more water. Now pee. Nap! Eat some more bread. I thought about my booze-soaked "intern week," which must have occurred right after I got pregnant.

I was already failing motherhood. It became a recurrent sentiment in my daughter's first year of life. Breastfeeding and pumping were more difficult than I had predicted. We used store bought formula and baby food. She developed a taste for Mac N Cheese. As a resident, I didn't know our pediatrician.

A few years passed. I did some growing.

I have a good friend, an Ivy-league educated attorney, who wants nothing more than to home school her children. I have another friend who posts on her [Facebook] page links to articles about the treacherous and unregulated world of daycare (the most recent was about a home daycare that burned down) or an admonition to her baby group that, really, if breast feeding was that hard our species would have died out eons ago. These are both woman I like and respect very much.

(continued)

R. Sweeting, MD (✉)
Division of Surgical Oncology and Endocrine Surgery, Department of Surgery,
Vanderbilt University, 597 PRB, 2220 Pierce Ave, Nashville, TN 37232, USA
e-mail: raeshell.s.sweeting@vanderbilt.edu

© Springer International Publishing AG 2018
K. Chretien (ed.), *Mothers in Medicine*,
https://doi.org/10.1007/978-3-319-68028-6_3

In my first year of motherhood, these things would have bothered me. Why didn't I want to home school? (And believe me, I don't.) Am I putting my children at risk in daycare? Is my daughter going to be fat, sick, and anti-social because I didn't [breastfeed] for 12 months? Was she already missing out on activities that would prove pivotal to her future success because I wasn't around to shuttle her from one to the other?

Of course not.

It took some time to become comfortable in motherhood, which itself has been the most intense and important undertaking in my life. That being said, I've come to realize that, for me, the Perfect Mom is not the Total Mom. I don't have a cohesive philosophy on motherhood save that the vast majority of us seem to be trying as best we can, and how we implement our universally held good intentions is both personal and family-specific. In regards to home schooling, prolonged [breastfeeding], nanny-care, organic this that and the other, epidurals, music appreciation class - they are all part of a decision making process that is individual to your family and lacking in any specific moral imperative.

For me and my family, it's best that I work. Aside from the obvious financial implications, work is good for me. I enjoy what I do and I choose to believe my children benefit from having a mother who feels this way about her vocation, even if it means daycare and formula and dinners on-the-fly.

I am not perfect. I get cranky, irritable, and short with people, some of them my off-spring, who deserve my patience. I don't think this makes me a bad mom, I think it makes me a human being. I gave up perfect a long time ago.

Although, all things being equal, I wish I hadn't drank during the first few weeks of my pregnancy...

—the red humor, "No such thing as perfect," May 3, 2013.

Many mothers in medicine start their journey of motherhood during residency, and there are challenges associated with being a mom during the rigorous years of residency. This chapter focuses on addressing some of those challenges and offering actionable advice as well as encouragement.

I began reading the Mothers in Medicine website during my intern year. I wasn't a mom yet, but I was a married female surgery resident. I knew I wanted to be a mom someday, but the idea of attempting this feat during residency seemed unthinkable. Then I found this remarkable community of women to help see me through.

I became a mother in medicine during my third year in residency. I actually found myself suddenly pregnant at the end of my second year—a year before my perfectly planned pregnancy goal and a year before my planned time in the lab. I scrambled, got into the lab a year early, and made it work. I spent most of my pregnancy, and first year of motherhood, working in a basic science lab. When my daughter was a year and a half, it was back to the grind of surgical residency. I found myself filling lots of roles at once. I was a more senior resident on the wards. My first intern was a newly minted mom of two. I felt a responsibility to support her and show her that we could do this together. My daughter visited me when she had barely seen me awake for days; my intern's husband brought her baby to meet us in the hospital coffee shop for quick kisses. We both managed to breastfeed. Speaking of which, I breastfed psychotically. It was the one thing I felt I could control.

Whenever I got home at night, it was the one untouchable bond I had with my little nugget. We lasted 2 and a half years—one of my proudest residency accomplishments. By the end of residency, my daughter had become a fixture in resident life. Days before my residency graduation, my little four-year-old peanut told me she wanted to be a surgeon when she grows up. I hold tight to this moment, her beautiful, joyful smiling face—as evidence that this is worth it and that she is gaining something from growing up with a mother in medicine.

Uncharted Territory

> *I feel quite isolated as the only resident in my male-dominated program to be a new mother/ pregnant in a long time, and at a hospital system where few female residents are mothers/ get pregnant during residency, in general.*
>
> *—Anonymous, "MiM Mail: A hard pregnancy during residency," February 8, 2016*

You don't have to go back far in history to find women who were asked about birth control on residency interviews. However, thanks to the sacrifices of generations of women before us, women now comprise nearly 50% of medical school classes [1]. Fields historically thought of as "male dominated" are seeing a change in demographics. Additionally, medical training often occurs when women are in their 20s and 30s. The age of medical students and residents has also been on the rise, with the average age of entering allopathic students currently at 24 and 26 for osteopathic students [2]. As a result, many women find themselves starting a family during residency. Despite many changes in the field of medicine, entering motherhood during residency can still feel like uncharted territory.

There Is Never a Good Time

> *My general takeaway regarding the subject of timing babies in medical training is that there is no perfect time. Each time is good in some respect and not so great in others. Having spent my 20s in pursuits of degrees, I didn't want to wait until I had a 'real doctor job.'*
>
> *—Mrs MD PhD, "Money and mothers in medical training," October 10, 2016*

There's never a perfect time to have a baby. This is a common aphorism expressed by parents in many professions and residency fits that sentiment perfectly. To speak about this honestly, there are significant challenges to having a child during residency. Recognizing these limitations and potential problems up front can help in getting through pregnancy and having a child. There are the physical demands of residency, such as minimal sleep and sometimes prolonged standing, which may make pregnancy more challenging. Ensuring adequate hydration and diet are also harder in residency when many are already struggling with basic self-care.

Additionally, time off in residency invariable affects many other people, as call structures are reliant on specific numbers of available residents. One approach for limiting the collateral effect on other residents is trying to plan so that the end of your pregnancy occurs during minimal call rotations or front loading your call in the second trimester. For women in residencies that include time for research or obtaining an additional degree (MPH, MBA, etc.), it can be helpful to attempt to have your child during these years. You may have more flexibility with maternity leave without the same impact on coresidents or your personal residency requirements. It is important to talk to your GME office early to discuss how maternity leave, FMLA, and extended time off are handled. There is significant variability among residency programs regarding maternity and family leave. Knowing the policies up front will help prevent you from unwanted extended residencies or disruptions to residency completion.

The strict leave policies in residency regarding time away from clinical rotations present a unique challenge to women in training. These challenges will not be solved with simple changes to maternity leave due to variability of individual certifying boards in each specialty. Although there is recognition that there is a need for better solutions, the problem of leave time remains [3].

The best way to prepare for having children in residency is to try and pick a supportive residency program from the beginning. Hopefully, someday this will be true of all residency programs, but the reality is that this is just not the case. One pediatric program director clearly makes the importance of family a known priority in his program.

> Make it clear the program is supportive in honoring reproductive choices or happenings, and our first concern is the health and well-being of parents and babies. You also make it clear that the resident's needs around child birth will not compromise or change the training of other residents, so all can celebrate the event.

> -Dr. Edwin Zalneraitis, Pediatric Residency Program Director,
> University of Connecticut.

If you can identify this type of supportive program on the front end, it will significantly help in providing you with the highest level of professional support to balance with your personal needs.

A common theme among program directors is the need for early communication. The earlier the program is aware, the easier it can be to arrange schedules in a way to allow for appropriate leave while minimizing effect on the new parent and other residents. In my case, my early communication with my scheduling chief and my program director allowed me to identify a mentor and transition to the lab a year early. A key component of being able to communicate early was my trust in my chief resident and program director to both work hard to find the best option while respecting my privacy about my early pregnancy. To illustrate the value of communication, Dr. Kathryn Andolsek, a program director in Family Medicine, mentioned that pregnancy is one of the few reasons for prolonged leave that can actually be planned during residency, unlike sudden illness or injury. Just as residency programs make arrangements in case of emergency leave, programs can make maternity leave work.

However, there are some realities of becoming a parent during residency that don't have ideal answers. One program director mentioned that as a parent, her desire to feel excitement for her residents is overshadowed by the real understanding that despite her efforts, this will be difficult. It is not possible as a program director to truly prepare a resident for the difficulties that lie ahead. Particularly for first-time mothers, there is just no way to truly anticipate the physical and emotional changes of motherhood, and the reality of the training environment is just not ideal. This is especially true when long, physically demanding call schedules is an unavoidable reality. Residency alone can push trainees to emotional limits, and motherhood does the same; the combination can be daunting. In summary, try your best to plan and work with your program but realize that many things will be out of your control.

Finding Your Army

It takes a village...and my village includes a housecleaner, a nanny, a back-up part-time nanny for on-call days, an amazingly flexible husband who works from home and one amazing non-medical friend I've made in this new city. Plus, in really important crunch times, a family willing to fly across the country for weeks at a time to care for my family. I come from a family whose resources definitely did not allow for hiring nannies or housecleaners, so I always feel a little self-conscious about it and hesitate to seek help, even when I know it's needed.

—*Ley, "Guest post: It takes a village," October 29, 2014*

If you have children during residency, it helps to build an army to help you raise your child. Many residents live in places in which they have no family available. Creating a village of help around you becomes essential. However, residency is time-consuming, making it difficult for residents to utilize and be familiar with local avenues for finding help. Residency does not lend itself to creating relationships outside of work that can help with childcare, nor does it provide you with the financial means to pay for an army. This creates real and difficult challenges to finding help and backup systems. As a result, it is necessary to capitalize on any and all opportunities to expand your sources of help.

Ways to Find Childcare/Backup Care

Ask your pediatrician about recommendations for childcare, nannies, backup care. Your pediatrician can be an amazing resource for trustworthy options. Occasionally, nurses are willing to provide childcare on their off days. Some institutions have an internal list of those willing to provide care. If not, you can usually ask around and find out who is willing to help. These are people you trust and people who also have CPR certification. Look to see if your hospital provides any reduced cost childcare/ backup care.

One of the unique challenges to the resident "army of support" is limited financial resources. When a small group of resident moms were polled about challenges of motherhood in residency, many cited the prohibitive costs of childcare in addition to the lack of convenient options. Many felt they needed more services to such as nannies, or housecleaning, but could not afford these with the added cost of a baby. While there are some hospitals with subsidized, onsite daycare, this still is not the norm. Despite a handful of studies done in the last few decades demonstrating increased productivity associated with onsite childcare, there is significant room for improvement [4, 5].

In addition to finding your army at home, it is important to find your support army at work. A wonderful study conducted by the Department of Medicine at the University of Missouri sought to recognize the growing needs of resident parents and to identify solutions to improve resident support. Their study demonstrated that although there is room for improvement, there are institutions who seek to support residents with families. [6] Seek out mentors you trust within your own institution. You will need people in your court. Find people who recognize your commitment to your work and your family and can help you nurture both.

As a surgery resident in a city without family with a working spouse in a demanding field, I found identifying support hard. Slowly, but surely, we created a little army, but it was daunting, and the honest truth is that I did a lot of crossing my fingers and praying that my daughter didn't get sick during stretches when I knew we didn't really have a good backup plan. It was hard, it put significant strain on my husband's job, and he clearly made unanticipated professional sacrifices as a result. But, we made it through and made a few lifelong friends in the process.

Mommy Guilt

As all working mothers do, I beat myself up daily for my inability to have it all and have a shred of energy left; I resent a society that reveres "perfect motherhood" while being unable to define what that is and unwilling to support it with policies that make sense for all mothers, working or not; I sometimes resent myself for my inability to be satisfied with "just" raising the children--why do I have to be a surgeon, of all things?--and then I have to laugh, because for this gender-role bending sworn feminist, the idea that one could be jealous of the stay at home side seems preposterous. But it's there.

—Wannabe WCW, "Hello from Paris," June 18, 2016

Be Prepared for Mommy Guilt

A group of resident moms were polled about difficulties in raising kids during residency. Each resident listed "mommy guilt" at some point in their responses. Guilt about being gone frequently, guilt about being exhausted when they are home, guilt about missing things at daycare or school, guilt about breastfeeding or not breastfeeding, working while home, or staying late to finish work at the hospital—this list goes on and on. But we are not alone in mommy guilt. It seems to be an universal problem [7]. Entire books have been devoted to the fight against mommy guilt [8–10].

The most important take-away is that you just need to keep going. Our society has created a completely unattainable picture of motherhood with none of the support needed to achieve it. Many of our policies and cultural practices do not value women or families. Ultimately, there are many different ways to raise children and many different ways to model parenting. You may not have as much time to offer, but when you have time, find ways to make it matter. Don't set yourself up for failure by planning and expecting extravagant days off. Just hang out, be silly and love on your kids. That's all that really matters to them. You will be surprised at how much kids just treasure their time with you even if you think it's not enough.

Breathe In and Out

Recently, I have been having a me-time problem. The problem is, I don't have any. Now, there are pressing and non-modifiable external reasons for my lack of a life, namely residency, which severely limits the total number of hours that I can devote to non-work activities. Then there is parenthood and I know I don't have to go into detail here at MiM about the ways in which that limits me-time. Let's just say: Last weekend I turned on the shower and read a New Yorker article while sitting on the bathroom floor and telling my daughter through the door in a sing-song voice that I was almost do-one with my show-er. So my expectations in the me-time department are not lofty.

—m, "The me-time problem," October 25, 2013

You will get overwhelmed. Being a resident is overwhelming. Being a mom is also overwhelming—put the two together and it won't be easy. So, don't forget self-care. I was once at an afterwork function when one of my mentors (who also has kids) noticed I was not fully breathing. I literally was too stressed to fully inhale and exhale. She rescued me, sat me in a chair, sent my husband home with my daughter, gave me a glass of wine, and said "Breathe in and breath out." Don't forget to breathe. Take a moment for yourself even if it's a few minutes on the way home or rocking out to your favorite song in the car.

I always found that the less I was taking care of myself, the more frazzled and overwhelmed I felt. My personal strategy for me-time was stopping at the Kroger on the way home from the hospital and just walking around for 10 min to decompress. I would often call and catch up with my mom on those walks as she has always been my most effective calming elixir. My grocery walks allowed me to feel centered when I walked into the house. It allowed me to shed just a little of the energy of the day. And, although the feeling of calm was usually fleeting (since reality swiftly creeped back in), it gave me a little foothold of control…and it helped us to have groceries!

"Don't Hide Your Kids"

The instructions to hide my daughter came from a good place. It came from an attending who had my best interest in mind. He mentioned that in this world even though I was working just as hard, family issues were going to be looked down upon. I would be stereotyped. People aren't used to mom surgeons, especially not as residents. He told me a story about sneaking off from work as a fellow to pick up his sick son by making up some elaborate story to hide the reason that he had to leave. "It is more respectable to meet friends for beer than try and pick up your child from daycare," he told me. My response…I would talk about my child incessantly! I figured, if the world wasn't ready for women to be both surgeons and moms, than I would help to make them ready.

—Cutter, "(Don't) Hide your kids!" August 8, 2014

This one is about change. Women in residency are part of the norm now. Women make up large percentages of residency programs across all specialties. As a result, mothers in residency are becoming a common occurrence. In order to shape the experience of mothers in residency and fight for appropriate leave policies and family support, it will become imperative to normalize the experience of mothering in residency. Dr. Zalneraitis wrote about his program, "We have a 90 day extension of full salary and benefits on short term disability if the OB says the parent is not ready to return. We have priority access to the University day care for residents. We have private, comfortable breast milk pumping areas with professional grade pumps and residents are relieved from duty when they need to pump. The University will extend compensation and benefits for any additional time needed." We should want these protections for all moms and must work to find ways to support moms while also preserving the overall experience of residency and the residency program.

Finally, as a mother in medicine, be a resource to other resident moms. Don't be afraid to mention the name of your child. If it is important to you, then bring your kids to social events. Nothing will ever change if we hide in the shadows.

We Have Something to Offer

It has changed me. Immensely. I know that I am so much more of a better clinician because of it. It keeps me up when I'm on call. It makes me teach the Interns and Medical Students more about how to care for our patients with all that we have. It makes me spend extra time reading and enhancing my knowledge base. It helps me give practical advice to my clinic patients and even though some families still can't believe I'm old enough to be a doctor, they seem more comforted when I talk to them about my own family.

I'm different because of this shining little boisterous boy who chose me to be his Mama. The one who drools on me as I laugh. The one who says "Mama go to work" and walks me to the door in the morning. I leave each day with him blowing me a kiss after I ask "dame un besito". He has given me this big 'ole fierce mama heart that I am soo thankful for. Most importantly, children are pretty amazing, and so are moms!

—Mommabee, "My Big 'ole Fierce Mama Heart," March 3, 2014

Being a mother in residency and in medicine in general is extremely valuable. It will inform the way you care for patients. It will change the way you relate to other people on your team. It will change your priorities and the lens by which you view the world. The practice of medicine is about taking care of people and demonstrating empathy, understanding, and knowledge. Being a mother is a valuable part of who you are as a resident physician.

My residency baby is now 6 years old. She is always happy, bright, energetic, and beautifully inquisitive. She still wants to be a surgeon (and a teacher, cowgirl, princess, scientist) and delights in asking me about my day. We all survived residency intact and strong—despite the bumps along the way.

Special acknowledgments to the many resident moms and residency program directors who shared their experiences with me.

References

1. Lautenberger DM, Dandar VM, Raezer CL, et al. The state of women in academic medicine. Washington: AAMC; 2013.
2. Age of applicants to U.S. Medical Schools at anticipated matriculation by sex and race/ethnicity, 2013-2014 through 2015-2016. AAMC. 2015.
3. Jagsi R, Tarbell NJ, Weinstein DF. Becoming a doctor, starting a family—leaves of absence from graduate medical education. N Engl J Med. 2007;357:1889–91.
4. Cotton D. Workplace day care: benefits to the employer. Dimens Health Serv. 1983;60(7):16–7.
5. Lehrer EL, Santero T, Mohan-Neill S. The impact of employer-sponsored child care on female labor supply behavior: evidence from the nursing profession. Popul Res Policy Rev. 1991;10:197.
6. Morris L, Cronk NJ, Washington KT. Parenting during residency: providing support for Dr Mom and Dr Dad. Fam Med. 2016;48(2):140–4.

7. George D. Despite "mommy guilt," time with kids increasing. Washington Post Staff Writer. Tuesday 20. 2007. p. A01.
8. Bort J, Pflock A, Renner D. Mommy guilt: learn to worry less, focus on what matters most, and raise happier kids. New York: AMACOM Division American Management Association; 2005.
9. Douglas S, Michaels M. The mommy myth: the idealization of motherhood and how it has undermined all women. New York: Simon and Schuster; 2005.
10. Rubin R. Despite potential health benefits of maternity leave, US lags behind other industrialized countries. JAMA. 2016;315(7):643–5.

Chapter 4
Being a Mother in Medicine in Practice

Monique Tello

> *I was 5 weeks pregnant and working in the spine room. Just as I finished my intubation and secured the airway, I turned to set the ventilator and administer some important medications. The surgery fellow started to position the fluoroscope near the patient's cervical spine, about a foot away from where I was working. "Please don't use the X-ray right now; I need to put on a lead shield first," I said. "Yeah, ok... whatever..." he said, as he continued to fine-tune its position. Thirty seconds later he sighed, then started pushing some buttons and eyeing the screen. I looked at him sternly and said, "I'm serious. Don't do it. I'm pregnant." After coos and congratulations from the fellow, resident, nurse, and scrub tech, I felt a bit awkward. Of course, I myself had just learned of my pregnancy; I hadn't even seen a heartbeat on ultrasound yet! This wasn't the way I expected to tell people my good news, and I really wish I hadn't been forced to do so in that situation. That being said, I really didn't want the radiation exposure at that time. I suffered a miscarriage a few weeks later and then had to engage those same people in some very awkward conversations.*
>
> —Dawn Baker, M.D., "Pregnant in the OR: When to tell," June 15, 2015

We all want to be good doctors *and* mothers, but I bet we've all asked ourselves how on earth that can happen. I have, anyways, when I've stumbled up our back steps at almost 7 p.m. on a weeknight herding two overtired and wired kids, balancing my work bag, kids' backpacks and lunchboxes, my coffee mug from the morning, and the house keys... and then my pager goes off. I know I've been waiting for an

M. Tello, MD, MPH (✉)
Massachusetts General Hospital/ Harvard Medical School,
55 Fruit Street, Yawkey 4B, Suite 4700, Boston, MA 02114, USA
e-mail: drmoniquetello@gmail.com

© Springer International Publishing AG 2018
K. Chretien (ed.), *Mothers in Medicine*,
https://doi.org/10.1007/978-3-319-68028-6_4

interpretation on a CT scan, and that page is the radiologist who will tell me if my patient has a bad thing going on in her belly. I need to answer them, understand the result, come up with a plan, and then call my patient.

But I also need to get these hungry monsters into the house, set some kind of healthy dinner in front of them, and keep them distracted, or I won't be able to close the loop on this case. I'm thinking: *How on earth can I do it all?*

Thriving in medicine and parenthood is possible, but there is no one-size-fits-all strategy. What works for me may not work for someone else. My life is full of variations of the above, and I've found that yogurts, raisins, and pretzels thrown on trays and set in front of some educational children's cartoon programming work wonders. Very fast, decently nutritious, acceptable entertainment, quiet children, case closed.

But what about for the surgeon-mom, the hospitalist-mom, the researcher-mom, the radiologist-mom... What kinds of situations do they have to navigate? How do we all manage to not only do our jobs, but also to excel and advance in our careers, and raise kids to become happy, well-adjusted good citizens? Our two worlds constantly overlap and intertwine and even collide. Is there a guide for this stuff?

Clearly, we here at Mothers in Medicine are trying to help. But ultimately, you are your own guide.

Yes, that sounds cheesy, but it is true: Only you can determine what your goals are as a physician and as a mom. I can't overstate this enough: No one can excel in a job if they aren't sure what they are supposed to accomplish. In any major quality improvement project or research study, the biggest question is: *What are the outcome measures?*

What are your basic career and family aspirations? Some physicians yearn to be a department chair or division chief, CEO of a hospital, or medical school dean. Others are fulfilled in small private practice, part-time clinical work, or 40-hour workweek shifts. Some feel best leaving clinical medicine behind to work in consulting, pharmaceutical development or public health. It's all good, as long as it's good for you.

What's most important for your kids, in your eyes: safety and security, health and wellness, and psychological stability? Do you want more than that: the best schools, world travel, and amazing experiences? Or proximity to loving family, meaningful engagement in a religious community, and many friends? How about all of the above?

For me, after spinning my wheels going in different directions (and, I admit, a lot of therapy), I figured out that I wanted to work in an academic medical center as a part-time clinician and educator, plus raise my kids within a nurturing community of family, friends, and neighbors. I'm very thankful that I have been able to live this dream.

Of course, what works for me may not work for you. The logistical advice in this chapter is designed to be a helpful jumping-off point. You may come to different conclusions, and that is totally fine. If you find other solutions that make you and your family happy, then congratulations!

Pregnancy

When to Tell?

When I was pregnant, it never occurred to me not to tell people. I can't keep a secret to save my life. But I have colleagues who kept their bumps hidden for as long as humanly possible, for many different reasons: worries about discrimination; fears of being passed over for promotion; superstition. I believe this is a personal decision, for the most part. However, our colleagues in radiology and in the operating room (as seen in the opening blog excerpt) often don't have the choice:

> *I had to disclose I was pregnant because I was a radiology resident. They had already made the schedule for upcoming residency and I noticed I was on fluoroscopy rotations during my pregnancy and for that reason, I had to disclose so they could rearrange the schedule.*
>
> *—Geri Chang, M.D.*

Others may have the option to delay disclosure, but choose to tell anyways:

> *I was pregnant as a 3rd year resident in a neurosurgery program. I didn't feel as if I had to hide it and informed everyone very early on. My fellow residents were not at all supportive, but I expected that. We are around a lot of X-ray exposure, but this never bothered me because lead blocks X-rays. I wore lead religiously in the OR and in the resuscitation room, so it was never an issue.*
>
> *—GCS15*

> *I did not hide any of my pregnancies- disclosed somewhere between 8 & 12 weeks with each in part for workplace protection- those who are pregnant get pregnancy radiation badges which helps to monitor exposure and also helps make others aware- most people were supportive of avoiding or at least limiting radiation exposure when not overly burdensome to do so. Also, my hospital's policy is that pregnant employees don't care for patients in droplet precautions... working mostly in a pediatric setting for two of my three pregnancies, it made sense to disclose early to limit my risk of having to take one of these patients to the OR where there would most certainly be exposure to whatever respiratory illness they had. For the most part, when pregnant I was not assigned to interventional radiology or the cardiac catheterization lab. Radiation exposure from c-arm in the OR is miniscule to zero for the anesthesiologist (especially if I moved myself as far back as I could get), so I was assigned to those rooms throughout (and I didn't honestly object). It was never a problem.*
>
> *—Rebecca Hong, M.D.*

If you do feel that you have a choice here, do consider: If you lose the pregnancy, would you want to have the support of anyone in particular? Maybe it would be just your partner, a best friend, close family members… Or, maybe you would want colleagues and supervisors to know.

Just 8 weeks into my first pregnancy, I had some bleeding. Of course I was seeing patients at the time, and I got through my clinic session before calling my OB/GYN, who saw me right away. The ultrasound revealed a small subchorionic hemorrhage, but we truly did not know if the pregnancy would be viable. Our OB/GYN was very guarded.

I decided to let my office know, not only because I had to keep running over to the OB office for scans, but also because I knew that if we lost the pregnancy, I would want to have a few days off. Our clinic is made up of female attendings and almost all-female staff, and it's a very supportive environment, which helps.

Of note, the pregnancy went to term, and he is now our seven-year-old boy!

In the end, when to tell (and who to tell) can be dictated by occupational demands or a very personal decision.

Managing Pregnancy Symptoms at Work

Pregnancy is not an illness. It's usually a joyful time in one's life. But man, can it make you feel awful. Morning sickness, fatigue, swelling, brain fog... Everyone experiences these things differently, but almost everyone is going to have something. Rare is the mom who can rosily exclaim, "Gee, I felt *wonderful* throughout my entire pregnancy!"

Even in the same person, pregnancy can present differently. With my first, I had very little nausea; rather, I had weird intense cravings for salty things (like sardines). So, when I learned I was pregnant with my second, I went out and bought cans and cans of sardines. Surprise! Not only did the mere whiff of sardines make me nauseated, that's how I felt for the whole 9 months.

Morning sickness, which, in my experience, can last all day and can be any variation on the same theme: vague queasiness, frank nausea, intermittent "burps," and projectile vomiting... I have friends who required admission and PICC lines for hyperemesis gravidarum.

If your nausea is manageable, ginger tea and Zofran can help. Ginger tea is sold commercially, but you can make your own with fresh ginger slices steeped in boiling water and sweetened with honey. (FYI, this concoction is a wonderfully effective home remedy for dyspepsia in general, IMHO.) Common sense approaches like eating very small yet frequent meals are key, for both morning sickness as well as the reflux that can develop toward the end of pregnancy. There's only room for so much in there... Calcium carbonate chewables can help with mild, intermittent reflux, but many will go on to require daily ranitidine. Why outline specifics here? Because whether you've got outpatient clinic or a busy O.R. schedule, you have to get through your day, darnit.

There's more than GI nastiness that can hinder the workday. In her bestselling book *Lean In*, Sheryl Sandberg won my heart when she described her massive weight gain and painfully swollen legs during her pregnancies. She suffered a great deal and very much appreciated the company's "pregnancy parking spaces" close to the building. In both of my pregnancies, I was driving in to the city and parking at a lot about a mile from the main hospital campus. That fifteen minute waddle was so incredibly painful, but it was also the only exercise I got for months on end. (I did manage to finagle "pregnancy parking" toward the end of my first pregnancy, which was in the heat of summer, and I was so incredibly grateful.)

Compression stockings or hose can be your friend here. I would tell you that there are attractive styles of compression garments nowadays, but there aren't. Let's face it, when your legs look like tree trunks, fashion takes a hit. While you're flaunting the granny gear, you might as well wear comfortable shoes, too. I traveled to work in Crocs flip-flops and then slipped into a cheap pair of oversized flats I picked up at a discount store. After pregnancy, when at least my feet and ankles went back to normal, I tossed the "fat" shoes. It felt good.

And of course, there's the fatigue, that deep, bone-weary, heavy fatigue of pregnancy: a hormonal cloud akin to pharmaceutical sedation. How I yearned to curl up under my desk, rest my head on my shoes, which I had taken off because my swollen feet hurt so much, and snooze. But, in the middle of a busy clinic day/full O.R. schedule/teaching conference, you just can't do that. Though caffeine intake can be associated with miscarriage, up to 200 mg daily has been deemed "safe." This is roughly the equivalent of a small, strong coffee from a certain Seattle-based chain cafe, FYI. Me? I drank about five cups per day throughout both pregnancies, and was still tired.

Don't want to risk any caffeine? A splash of cold water on the face, followed by a drink of the same can help. Revive and hydrate; this can temporarily "wake" things up. Go ahead, drink up—you're going to have to pee anyway. Of course, if insomnia is an issue, as it so often is, even a Polar Plunge into the nearest body of water during winter isn't going to wake you up. Sleep apnea, reflux, and frequent urination: it all conspires to limit your restful slumber.

Later in pregnancy, as that big belly stretches and weakens the core muscles, many aches and pains can set in. Unless you're one of those super-doc-moms who can maintain a regular yoga or Pilates practice the whole 9 months, you're likely to suffer from something. Very commonly, it's sacroiliac (SI) joint dysfunction. I describe this as feeling like one of the bones in the low back is just slightly out of place, and if you could just snap it back, you'd feel sooo much better... and this is not far from the actual pathology. There are a number of stretches designed to realign the sacrum and pelvis, but formal physical therapy can be a godsend. If you have time.

What do other mothers in medicine have to say about their pregnancy symptoms?

Pregnancy...oh boy. My baby turns 1 tomorrow. I'm pondering a second...What symptom didn't I have? 7 months of nausea - struggled with it for the first 12 weeks of pregnancy, then I couldn't take it any longer and took Diclegis which helped a ton. Could only eat carbs for the first trimester.

Burning tummy in the middle of the night - kept muffins on my night table. SI joint dysfunction - started week 16, couldn't walk more than 1-2 blocks at a time. It improved after delivery, but I couldn't get back to my regular running routine. Eventually I went to PT and with some hip flexor/psoas stretches it improved. Insomnia - second and third trimester. Would be awake from 1-4AM for 3 nights, then crash and sleep through the night for one night. Around this time, my clinic tried to increase my work hours. I ended up going on FMLA (using 1 hour per day) in order to continue with my regular clinic schedule. Lower extremity swelling, a little gingivitis, acne, reflux, poor memory....I think I've forgotten the rest of the symptoms, LoL.

—*Working girl, January 19, 2017*

Intense skin itching necessitating 3am Aveeno baths (it worked!) with daughter. Bad back acne with my daughter requiring erythromycin. Reflux required prescription (at the time) Prilosec with daughter. Nausea so bad in first trimester with son I had saltines and Andes mints on hand constantly at work to try to prevent dry heaving at the scope (luckily no throwing up and I usually made it to the stairwell to dry heave alone). I had SI joint dysfunction also that became tear inducing after a week of bedrest when my son came early and required intense chiropractic work to recover. Nightly leg cramps, I guess due to electrolyte imbalance, that would wake me up in intense pain - I researched a physical foot stretch maneuver to extinguish the cramps. In our field of work, and society, we are taught to push through it, but it's not for the faint of heart.

—Gizabeth Shyder, January 23, 2017.

I had intense sacro-iliac and pubic symphysis pain. I also got severe spasms of my piriformis and related muscles in compensation which was painful. My first pregnancy, when I was a fellow, I borrowed a wheeling stool and did most of the rounds sitting on it moving from outside room to room. I only stood up when we were actually in the patient rooms, and sat during all the presentations and plans (which took most of the time) as well as scooting myself between rooms. My second pregnancy it got much worse and I was in private practice, so I just swallowed my pride and used a cane everywhere outside of exam rooms. I did physical therapy both times but honestly, it didn't do much in either case until after I delivered, in which case it worked great to get me back to my normal self. I also had horrible reflux, to the point in my second pregnancy where I would awaken at night panicked with half digested food feeling like it was in my airway. One night I actually apparently aspirated something because I woke up suddenly very SOB I had incredible SOB and CP and wheezing for days afterwards (yes, I did see my OB). I ended up having to take Zantac, sleep on a significant incline, and eat and drink nothing at all after 6 PM, as well as cut out anything spicy or tomato based or too greasy. Milk was really my friend during that time.

—Dad3Mass, January 24, 2017

Occupational Health Concerns

Doctors are potentially exposed to radiation and chemicals in the line of duty, and this brings up very specific concerns in pregnancy. Those in the operating room and the cath lab have to consider and mitigate these issues. Below are the views from anesthesiology and cardiology:

Pregnant in the Operating Room

Regardless of your position, occupational hazards exist when working in the operating room. Normally these things aren't given too much thought, but when my choices suddenly affected another developing life, it caused me to pause and contemplate these hazards on a deeper level. Unfortunately, studies on pregnant healthcare workers (and other occupations) are difficult to interpret due to the fact that they predominantly consist of retrospective cohort data rife with selection and recall bias or animal studies of direct exposure to substances. Nevertheless, here is a list of some things to consider when working pregnant in the operating room or hospital setting [1–3]:

Anesthetic Gases. *While every effort is made to avoid elective surgery during pregnancy, even pregnant women need to have general anesthesia under urgent circumstances; there is*

(continued)

no evidence that gases administered at concentrations appropriate for general anesthesia cause fetal harm. Thus, sub-anesthetic levels that would be passively inhaled in an occupational capacity should theoretically be safe as well. That being said, it is generally recommended that pregnant women in the OR avoid inhalation of the gases when possible. We facilitate this by using ventilator circuits with scrubbing systems and taking care to turn off anesthetic gases if the circuit is open to air for a period of time (such as between mask ventilation and intubation). This is mostly routine practice regardless of pregnancy status.

Methylmethacrylate. MMA is a common ingredient in cement mixtures for joint prosthetics. When mixed, it forms a strong scent which dissipates over a number of minutes as the mixture cures. Studies, which have mainly occurred in animal models, reveal mixed results in terms of impact on fetal development. As a pregnant provider, your choices are to not work on cases using MMA, ask the scrub mixing the cement to use a vacuum device to remove the fumes, or temporarily leave the room during the mixing process. In one human study, MMA was not found above a 0.5 ppm level in breast milk of surgeons who utilized vacuum mixing devices. At our institution, the use of these devices is mixed amongst surgery personnel, but local suction can also be easily employed. If I am in a joint room and my patient is stable, I elect to step into the adjacent substerile core (which has a window to the operating room) for a few brief minutes while the mixing occurs. However, I did have a recent case where the patient was very unstable and I could not leave the room or easily turn the case over to another provider temporarily. After that experience, the scheduler changed me to a different OR.

Radiation. Radiation is commonly used during OR procedures such as orthopedic repairs, gastrointestinal explorations, interventional pain management, interventional radiology, angiography, line placement... I could go on. For radiation, potential harmful effects are directly related to the dose of exposure. The CDC website has a table of radiation doses with corresponding maternal/fetal risks at different gestational ages. At doses higher than 50 rads, risks range from failure of implantation and miscarriage at early stages to growth retardation, mental delay, and increased risk of cancer at later stages. As with general anesthesia, pregnant women themselves must occasionally undergo irradiative procedures, but care is always taken to balance risks with benefits. In addition, protective shielding goes a long way to reduce exposure. Even in an occupational capacity we wear protective lead garments during periods of radiation. Wearing these and standing at least 6 feet away from the beam will decrease the exposure by more than 99%. However, the garments must encircle the body and not just cover the front of the body in apron form. This is especially important for anesthesiologists, who often turn their backs to the OR table to gather drugs or supplies, etc. And during my pregnancy, I have actively avoided assignments that involve continuous use of fluoroscopy (such as cath lab, GI lab, and interventional vascular or radiology).

Infection. It goes without saying that universal precautions need to be followed by everyone, but there are wider implications and possible sequelae if a pregnant woman contracts an infectious disease while working in the OR. Discussing the details of this would be beyond the scope of this article, but the gist is that potentially teratogenic effects of certain microbes and their treatments and/or long-term transmission of viral infections to the fetus such as HIV or HCV are considerations that should provide pause and vigilance when employing personal protection.

(continued)

Stress. This is the most difficult "hazard" to avoid. Theoretically, emotional and physical stress can cause neuroendocrine and cardiovascular alterations that could affect fetal physiology and hence possible outcomes. Limited studies implicate longer working hours, night shift work, prolonged standing, and physical work as risk factors for preterm birth, SGA infants and miscarriage. It must also be mentioned, especially for trainees, that the financial burden of NOT working during pregnancy can cause significant stress in itself. Some women might choose to take a lighter load or less frequent call shifts during pregnancy, if possible.... Vigilance to self-care post-call and adequate hydration during call can help.

—Dawn Baker, "Pregnant in the Operating Room," August 5, 2015

Pregnant in the Cath Lab

There is no harm in being protective of your unborn child. There is no harm in speaking up for yourself when you have strong feelings about any subject. For heaven sakes we are in a healing profession- we should take care of one another too. We should make a pact- all MiM and MiM followers to steadfastly protect and promote the (physical and mental) well being of our gravid counterparts.

First, to get this out of the way, there is a major difference between therapeutic (or diagnostic) radiation exposure vs. occupational radiation exposure. All physicians would consider using x-rays to examine or treat a pregnant woman, as long as the benefit outweighs the risk. Do you need dental xrays while pregnant? Probably not. If you have a serious condition during pregnancy requiring imaging, all attempts will be made to use alternative non-radiation imaging or to at least minimize fetal exposure. The risk to the fetus is based on amount of exposure (may vary based on type of exam) and week of pregnancy. It would be a mistake to x-ray a pregnant woman without considering the fetus (therefore the questions and signs in radiology). However, it is important to note that just because there are signs and attempts made to avoid exposure in no way means that it is absolutely contraindicated.

Here as Mothers in Medicine we are discussing occupational exposure: a classic intersection of personal responsibility and professional obligation with undercurrents of gender discrimination. We would all take a bullet (literally) for our children, our own safety/sanity is only a secondary concern. What are we willing to expose our children to: now that is a hot topic.

Fifty percent of Internal Medicine residents are women, yet only 14% of all cardiology fellows and a mere 7% of practicing cardiologists are women. We may be few, but as women in cardiology we are a serious bunch- and are concerned about why more women do not consider careers in cardiology. It is likely women are deciding not to pursue cardiology early- as medical students or interns. Concern over lifestyle and radiation exposure during mothering years is likely a key issue.

Tackling the subject head on, two important papers are published in cardiology journals. The first published in JACC in 1998 (http://www.ncbi.nlm.nih.gov/pubmed/9525565) is a consensus statement for radiation safety in the cath lab. This year another consensus statement (http://www.ncbi.nlm.nih.gov/pubmed/21061249) was published by a group of women interventional cardiologists (now these are women who I seriously admire). I recommend that you read both if this issue affects you directly.

(continued)

Here are important points I would like to make:

1. Fundamental radiation science: exposure is proportional to energy emitted, inverse to distance from source, and subtracted by protective equipment. When pregnant I wore two layers of lead (my usual apron) in my first trimester then special pregnancy apron (even though it weighed 12 lbs-or maybe a TON) the rest of the time. I never let the fellows control the fluoro pedal and when able always took an extra step away from the camera. On occasion I took it as an excuse to stay far, far away from the table, on a stool in the corner where I could rest my feet too, a bonus.

2. When I was a fellow one of my female attendings was pregnant. It really helped me to see her in this role. She gave me the best advice. Meet with the University Radiation Officer-this really helped to balance my fears with what is known about the risk.

3. The female fellows in my current program are not allowed to work in the cath lab during pregnancy. This takes the decision making away from them. I am not 100% behind this, only because it is really hard for them to find coverage for maternity leave already.

4. X ray is not the only source of radiation exposure. I learned from the Radiation Officer that my greatest risk would be during my nuclear cardiology rotation. Patients dosed with isotope emit radiation, and despite high standards areas of radiation can be present in the department. Always wear your badge when reading nuclear studies, do not leave your lunch in the reading room, and for heaven sakes, do not do injections for nuclear stress tests or PET scans.

5. The total amount of radiation allowed in pregnancy is 0.5 mSv per month and 5 mSv for entire pregnancy. This is 10% of the amount of radiation defined as negligible by ACOG guidelines (Obstet Gynecol 2004;104:647–651). Studies from diagnostic radiology in pregnancy show exposure below 50 mSv is not associated with fetal loss or anomaly. Other population studies suggest that exposure to 100% of the allowed radiation during pregnancy will increase the risk of having a child with congenital anomaly from 4.0% to 4.01%. The chance your child will develop cancer will increase from 0.07% to 0.11%.

6. It is difficult for me to compartmentalize my role as mother and cardiologist. It all runs together in an overwhelming way. Eight weeks pregnant, while taking progesterone for a fetus at risk, I was inches away from the camera while doing CPR on a woman while my partner inserted a temporary pacemaker. I had lead on, but had not yet declared my pregnancy and did not yet have a fetal badge. During my 2nd trimester I was exposed to acute viral myocarditis, amazingly three times where two of the three patients were killed. Suspected viruses can cause fetal hydrops. The surviving patient was a miracle and my ability to cure him was instrumental. My team knew I had ID consultation and special tests by Employee Health. They did not know I took a "time out" in the call room where I sobbed uncontrollably for 20 minutes.

I carried two pregnancies and worked in the cath lab both times. I checked my fetal badge religiously every month. Under my lead, over 18 months of pregnancy my fetal badge (s) summed total radiation exposure of <0.01 mSv, below the measurable limit, ZERO.

It is probable that women avoid their true calling into cardiology due to concern over the occupational hazard. It is possible those who do pursue cardiology still face additional obstacles based on current maternity policies (I think this is true of most of medicine). My experiences thus far have been challenging, and I hope we can make things better for the next generation.

For the sake of full disclosure, in addition to exposing both of my boys to radiation, I also ate lunch meat, non-pasteurized cheese and even drank a glass of wine (or two) during my third trimester.

—J.C., "Pregnant in the Cath Lab," May 11, 2011

As J.C. admits, I also ate lunch meat and non-pasteurized cheese and even drank a glass of wine (or two) in pregnancy. How would I personally feel about occupational radiation exposure? As an outpatient internal medicine attending, it's difficult for me to imagine. Here are some of the reader comments on these and related posts:

I refuse to inject intrathecal chemotherapy while pregnant. Not sure of the data either way, but it is my choice. In this situation, you get to do what you think is best. Enough said.

—The Red Humor, May 10, 2011

I'm in [pediatrics]. I also avoided going into isolation rooms with chicken pox patients, and avoided CMV and HSV patients. I return the favor now by seeing those patients, (doing all the viral swabs etc.) for the pregnant residents.

—Anonymous, May 10, 2011

I think we all have situations where risk is unavoidable and you just do your best. I was pregnant as an attending on a BMT ward. There really was no way for me to avoid HSV and CMV exposures because that would have meant not ever attending. So I did my best to use gown and gloves when I definitely knew or highly suspected. That said, if there was a way to avoid exposure, I did.

—Anonymous, May 10, 2011

Theoretically radiation is most worrisome during the period when there's a lot of growth and cells are dividing rapidly, ie in utero and childhood. I'd be a little anxious about malformations (warranted or unwarranted) but also worried/feeling guilty about the adding to the cumulative doses of radiation the kid would be getting and the lifetime effects. A little bit here, a little bit there… it adds up! I think you're right to protect the baby as much as possible.

—Anonymous, May 10, 2011

My feeling is that if you can avoid a risk, do so. I skipped coffee and its bad effects are dubious. I did have a fall with a broken ankle that required X-rays but felt awful about it.

During my residency we regularly stepped in for our colleagues. Of course those were the days of no days of and 120 hour weeks, so if you did not help each other you did not survive.

I do not know why people pooh-poohed your risk or your trying to avoid it. Aren't we supposed to put baby's health first?

—sunnid, May 10, 2011

Pregnant ortho resident here -- can't avoid it, really; I can't exactly refuse to do almost all cases on my current x-ray heavy rotation (trauma) so I wear a lead skirt and a full-length lead apron over top of that. (Plus thyroid shield.) It can get heavy and hot but it's manageable. And I'm ok with it. There have been three other residents recently in my program before me (with 5 babies between them during residency!) all with the same situation. All healthy babies. But that's just our little anecdotal n=5. :)

—Anonymous, May 10, 2011

Deliver at Your Own Hospital or Elsewhere?

When the provider is pregnant, there are other considerations. Do you want to be cared for at your own hospital? I could not have imagined going anywhere but the OB/GYN office down the hall from mine. My lovely OB was a clinical instructor in the same course as me, and I ran into her at the medical school from time to time, in between my prenatal appointments. She'd seen my hoo-ha and God knows what else down there on multiple occasions, and yet we would find ourselves standing around pleasantly chatting about curriculum changes while sipping lukewarm coffee. I didn't care.

Still, with my first, I went a little psycho around delivery. I created an annoying three-page natural-no-epidural birth plan with all sorts of stipulations: no medical students, minimal residents, and no male anybody. Any OB will tell you that the more controlling the mom-to-be is, the worse her delivery is going to be. It's Murphy's Law.

And so my first delivery was a disaster. Over forty-eight hours of labor. Transverse arrest. Fetal bradycardia. When the meconium hit the fan, there I was being wheeled into an O.R. crowded with every level trainee and both genders well represented. I didn't care. My son had to be rapidly and forcefully extracted during an emergency C-section: yanked from above and pushed from below. But he was born and he was healthy and all was good.

For my second, I had no plan. As a matter of fact, I was paralyzed. I was so traumatized by how violently *opposite* everything had turned out from what I had envisioned the first time around, I couldn't make any decisions at all. So my lovely OB firmly (but nicely) guided me through a successful VBAC (vaginal birth after C-section).

I've seen her around since, and we are very friendly. I've probably also run into multiple nurses, residents, and students who were witness to my howling hysteria in one or the other delivery, but I can't remember who was there from either so who cares. Personally, I'm glad that I delivered with a physician I know professionally and admire. I could never have managed going to any other hospital but my own anyways, too inconvenient.

But not everyone feels the same way. The question occurred to me: Where do pregnant doctors deliver? Is it different for OB/GYNs and anesthesiologists?

I posed the question to the Mothers in Medicine readers, and everyone who commented had a positive experience being in a familiar place surrounded by familiar people:

> *I also gave birth at the academic hospital where I work. I am an anesthesiologist and work in the OR with the couple of OB residents who helped deliver my baby, but I requested to have no OB medical students because I thought it would be awkward if I were ever to have them with me on their Anesthesia rotation. I also had a colleague attending do my epidural as opposed to an anesthesia resident for the same reason. Otherwise I felt like it was good to deliver in a familiar place with familiar faces.*
>
> —*PracticeBalance*

> *Anesthesia resident here! I chose to deliver at my hospital for insurance reasons, but I'm so glad I did. The OB residents treated me like family. I had a lot of pre-term contractions and would frequently drop by triage for a quick exam/US to make sure I wasn't in labor. They were wonderful! And I let one of my junior residents do my epidural when the time came- as residents, we do hundreds of these, so I had no problem letting a non-attending do it. The worst part? The OB status board displays your current weight/BMI... mortifying!!!! But so glad I delivered at my own hospital.*
>
> —*Anonymous*

> *I delivered my first at the small rural hospital where I work, by my OB/GYN colleague (I am FP with OB.) It was a wonderful experience. In the end my baby had to be shipped to a hospital 40 minutes away with a NICU. My second baby I delivered at said hospital with a*

NICU.... I had a great experience at that hospital as well. Were it not for complicated preg-
nancies and NICU stays, though, I would definitely choose to have them at my small hospi-
tal where everybody knows me and I felt loved and cared for.

—Emily

I am a family doc who does OB in a smaller town. I saw one of my female partners for my
prenatal care. I had a two day induction as I was post dates and we knew baby was big.
First day one of the female OBs was on; second day it was a male OB. I, of course, ended
up with a C-section after pushing for 3+ hours and said male OB was the one who did it.
At that point I did not care. The funny part with him is that he worked in the city where I
attended med school in a neighboring state and I worked with him on my OB rotation. It's
crazy how we ended up in the same small town. I work with him all the time and he did my
repeat C-section (during my first section he said "you're not going to want to VBAC next
time are you?") It was nice delivering in the hospital where I work and knowing the nurses
that were taking care of me. It never occurred to me to not deliver there.

—Rachel

Maternity Leave

How long should you take? How long *can* you take? Before my first delivery, I anticipated that I would want every second of my three-month maternity leave. My job allowed two months' paid leave and one month vacation time. I was very surprised when six weeks rolled around, and I couldn't wait to be back at work, or anywhere else: just out of the house.

I was one of the lucky ones. Not everyone gets three whole months without interruption of pay, and I am very thankful. But for my second, I definitely went back to work a couple of weeks early.

Everyone will be different on this front, but for those who felt or feel guilty that they'd prefer to get out of the house/interact with adults/be intellectually challenged/think about things other than pee, poop, and feeding, then you are not alone. I felt that way, and yes, I was always very glad to get home to snuggle with my little ones. Probably more glad than if I had just been at home all day, frankly.

Other doctor-moms write:

I was off for eight months (not entirely maternity leave - also leaving a job and starting a
practice.) That first day in the new office was exhilarating and fun. I didn't feel rusty; I felt
like I was back where I belonged. I HATED being home full-time

—Jay

I did not feel rusty at the end of my maternity leave (6 weeks, during which I wrote a case
report, took curbsides by e-mail and kept up with the literature.) But I certainly didn't feel
rested -- I felt edgy, bored out of my mind and unappreciated as a human being rather than
just a provider of milk. I actually wanted to return to work earlier, but my residency pro-
gram wouldn't let me. I've made it very clear to the chief of my division that if I ever have
another kid, I'm only going to take 2-4 weeks off, then come back 50% time for the rest of
my maternity leave. I think sitting at home with a baby for weeks is cognitively bad for me.

—Larvaldoctor

The flip side of this is that in the United States, many women are made to feel guilty for taking any maternity leave at all. The Family Medical and Leave Act of 1993 "entitles eligible employees of covered employers to take 12 weeks of unpaid, job-protected leave for the birth of a child, adoption, or foster child with continuation of group health insurance coverage under the same terms and conditions as if the employee had not taken leave." Despite this, bosses and colleagues may gripe about having to cover. There may be intense pressure to go back to work earlier than is planned, or than is healthy. Many of us have plenty to say about that:

> These stresses that new moms go through are not limited to medicine, but I think we are even more anxious because of our sense of responsibility to our patients and colleagues. This lack of respect and accommodation for motherhood is an endemic problem in the USA. Other western countries grant maternity leave to both fathers and mothers. France supports new moms for a year with nursing visits and job protection. Yes, we all wonder how they do it...but they do. As professional women we need to keep shining the light on the inequities we face and DON'T FEEL GUILTY for recovering from childbirth and spending precious time with our newborns. We are still pioneers in the workplace with the dual responsibility of being a mom and a doctor. It is not heresy to put family first and those precious baby moments are gone way too soon. (I feel a little tear welling up right now).
>
> —Dr. T.B.

> I am currently pregnant w/twins. These will be numbers 3&4. My first two children I had at my old job where several other mothers worked as well. There, everyone was very accommodating and helpful. I worked full-time up until the day I delivered in order to have a full maternity leave at home with my child. Now, I've changed jobs to a place where I'm the only mother. It's interesting to note the differences. I now work part-time and am salaried, and my medical director expects me to cover any emergencies on my days off with my patients (my previous job, we regularly covered the part-timers without a second thought). He has actually refused to help my nurse with critically abnormal labs on my days off, telling her to call me at home. Now that I have mentioned that I may be on extended leave secondary to my OB expecting to put me on bedrest at 32wks (you know, because of advanced maternal age AND twins), I am getting a huge amount of push-back. Although the clinic regularly employs locums physicians, my medical director has all but told me that I am to find my cover for this time as he doesn't plan on covering my patients. Truthfully, I'm already looking for job #3.
>
> —The Mommydoctor

> After my first maternity leave three years ago, one colleague who had her child years before FMLA, called me at home to suggest that I thank those who had covered my patients. As calmly as possible, I explained to her that our boss should be thanking her as it was the boss who had decided against spending the money to find coverage and that I was entitled to that time and therefore would be thanking no one.
>
> —Gizabeth Shyder

Breastfeeding/Bottle-Feeding (Because It's All Feeding)

I never in a gajillion years expected breastfeeding to be as hard as it was. Before my son's delivery, I had a prenatal lactation consult. I read not one, not two, but three books on breastfeeding. I bought the sterile plastic bags and freezer containers for all the milk I was going to pump before I went back to work.

But I struggled mightily. And then by two weeks into it, I couldn't wait to wean. I've written about this endlessly: it hurt. Oh my god, did it hurt. I had read about breastfeeding pain and pooh-poohed the accounts. *Those wussy moms*, I thought, smugly. But oh, did the world get its revenge on me for my judgment.

I was not alone, as I learned. Many other doctor moms struggle with breastfeeding and pumping, to the point that many conclude it's just not worth all the hassle:

I never pumped either. I breast fed the majority of my maternity leave. I hated breastfeeding. It caused me so much stress and guilt. As a resident, I don't have an office and our residency is very resident-run. Attendings are also passive aggressive. They wouldn't flat out tell me not to do it but it was just known that it's better to not do it. However, there was no place to pump. The pumping room was not even in the hospital. It was across the street on the undergrad campus—no one would let me take the time to walk over there and pump and do all that. So I pumped as much as I could during maternity leave and once I started work I pumped in the morning and evening for another month or two until my supply tanked. It was the best I could do in my current situation. If I had to do it again, I would relieve myself of the guilt and stress of it all. Chloe turned out just fine.

—Geri Chang

Pumping at work...what misery! I used every spare minute at work to pump for the first 2 months back with my first; then my pump broke while on in-house 30 hour call...I ended up having to tell my senior resident: sorry, but I have to go home (for spare hand pump parts) and I'll be back in 45 min....embarrassing! Facilities were totally not acceptable, shower of locker room, no privacy really at all. Decided to limit pumping to ~1/day (lunch only) after that and supplement with formula. This worked much better for me for another 3 months until I gave it up entirely. 2nd pregnancy, decided to do only 1x/day pumping again and supplement w/formula from the beginning; this worked well for me until baby was 10 months old. 3rd pregnancy, attempted to pump at work (1x/day), gave it up after 2 months... miserable and much more difficult as an attending as no guaranteed breaks in my day. If I am to have any more kids, plan to not pump at work at all...baby will be just fine w/formula and I will be a much less stressed mom and employee.

—Anonymous

Oy. Here's what I tell my patients. Breastfeeding actually is best for your baby (I usually try to suggest that it will help them lose baby weight, especially the younger ones) however I also tell them that only they can make the best decision regarding what is the best form of nutrition for their child. A bad mother is one that does not feed her baby at all. I breastfed my first child for 3.5 months and my second for seven months. Both times exhaustion and call schedule won out against milk supply, and it dwindled. Boy was I glad for formula, especially since I couldn't do as evolution intended and walk around with a child on the breast the entire day to stimulate milk supply. And yes, I got totally neurotic about how much I was pumping, blah blah blah. Never did store that much cause they ate it all! At any rate, when I got upset or obsessive, I tried to remind myself: Bad moms are ones that don't feed their babies period. Breastfeeding is HARD. Add a full time job where your first responsibility is supposed to be other people's well being and not your family's, and it's a super human feat.

—OB in NJ

I put these experiences up front to not only validate my mother-in-medicine colleagues whose experiences were less than optimal, but also to highlight the fact that *it's perfectly ok to formula feed*. Letting the whole breastfeeding/pumping thing go may, in the end, be the healthiest choice for a mom and her baby. That's personal, and if you are out there suffering, remember that it's *your* choice. Ignore any judgey nosy unhelpful opinions, and take strength from the shared experiences of your colleagues.

Of course, many working moms make breastfeeding and pumping work. I have great admiration for those who not only succeed at breastfeeding, but enjoy it. I am in absolute sheer awe of those who manage to pump at work. I never needed the private room and pumping ensemble in my clinic. Other moms rock this setup. How do they do it?

Many mothers in medicine offered their experience and advice in response to a post from pathologist Gizabeth Shyder titled "How To And Not Breast Pump At Work," and here is a compilation by topic:

Tips for Pumping

Planning Ahead

- *Make sure you introduce one bottle of pumped milk a day at around three weeks (this will help baby accept bottle and still take the breast). A colleague/friend of mine did this then slacked off right before she went back to work from three months of maternity leave - didn't do the bottle for a week. She went back to work and her daughter wouldn't take the bottle!*

Equipment

- *Do everything humanly possible to make pumping as easy as imaginable for you...as stated in the post, buy the more expensive dual pump*
- *I went through pumping twice, once as a resident, once as a solo-practitioner. Both times I purchased a new Medela "Pump in Style." Backpack style 1st go around, messenger bag style 2nd go around. (Oh, the exorbitant extravagance, I know, but when I got my old pump out of storage to clean up the second time around, it was, erm, moldy. Hence, brand new pump.) They were easy to take back and forth to work, came with a snazzy little milk cooler and freeze pack with little niches carved out for the bottles, and wonderfully efficient. With the dual pump I could be done pumping in 15-20 minutes, easily. Even nicer, I could always get extra pump parts from L&D storage because our hospital grade pumps were also Medela*
- *-Get a pumping band [or bra]...that way you can go handless and study or if you still have paper notes, do these during pumping...or, though it may make some shudder, even pump while driving if you have any sort of commute*
- *Additional tip- my best friend showed me how you can tuck the pump shield into your nursing bra (if left fastened) and go hands free without a band. I found this worked only with bras without underwire.*
- *If there are no pumps available for you to use at the hospital (such as one in the NICU or somewhere else in the hospital) consider buying a cheap pump to have at home and leaving a nice one in a locker at work so you don't have to lug the pump back and forth every day*
- *Agree with the pump 'bra,' I was able to type while pumping (though part of me wished I didn't have this option and could have just zoned out).*
- *My hospital has a rental program where I was able to keep a hospital grade pump in my office. I then had a standard model at home.*

Location

- *Talk to the lactation consultants in your hospital, they helped me discover pumping rooms (some with fridges) all across the hospital campus*
- *Do your research on what pumping facilities are available, how you will cover your patients while you are pumping, etc BEFORE you return to work, not on your first day back*
- *On L&D, we actually had so many nurses and staff nursing and pumping at the same time, we would designate a particular L&D room for "Fred" (the floor hospital grade pump) and any of us that wanted to would store our pumping things in that room and use it while on L&D.*

- *Having an office with a door that locks was very helpful. For those of you who are faculty members, think about helping your trainees find a safe comfortable place. Chances are they will not ask for special arrangements to be made for them.*

Pumping Schedule

- *Make sure you talk to someone in your specific field of medicine. I imagine anesthesiology has some unique challenges, since surgical cases are of variable length and it may take some specific planning to get a break to go pump.*
- *Just from talking to people and from my own experience, if you really want to keep your milk production up, it's a good idea to pump three times a day at least until six months. However don't feel badly if this isn't possible, just realize you will probably be supplementing with formula (which is not a failure in any way! Just something to be prepared for).*
- *I would nurse before I left the house, go round, pump in my office before morning patients, at lunch time, and around 3 pm (that session was the first to go, as my office staff could never manage to block a 30 minute window of time). When I got to go home (no labor patients.) I would either nurse Bean when I got home or pump if he had been fed recently.*
- *Luckily, OB/GYN is pretty darn supportive. It really rarely took more than 20 minutes [to pump] at any given stretch, so it wasn't like I was forever slacking on the work or anything. I more or less treated it like a really long bathroom break. It simply had to be done. I don't recall getting any flack...except for my office staff, who could not, for the life of them, remember to block 30 minutes in the 3 o'clock hour for me to pump (ok, so maybe I am bitter about this and need to let it go??)*

Pumping While on Call

- *I brought the pump with me, brought extra bottles, kept the microwavable steam bags (so awesome) in the pump bag, and kept my labeled bottles in the "milk fridge" on L&D (a nice commodity to have). I would pump every 3-4 hours and try to mimic my nighttime feeding schedule as closely as I possibly could.*
- *I would pump in the on-call room, aiming to pump every three to four hours. Sometimes, surgery or L&D would get hairy and I would get the "torpedo effect" as Gizabeth so beautifully describes. I cannot tell you the physical *relief* it is to pump after going so long!*
- *I didn't have a real problem with supply (thankfully!), but a pump can take some getting used to. I found it helpful to bring a picture of my baby with me, and look at it, or to imagine breastfeeding. It made it easier to get to the letdown reflex, and that can make pumping more comfortable and effective.*
- *I always thought of breast milk/nursing as the one thing I could do for my baby that no one else could, so that on those call nights or just long days when I wouldn't see him awake I had something to hold on to that made me feel a little less guilty about being a working mom*

Self-Care

- *[I breastfed] for four months, two months at work. I wished I could have gone longer. My milk dried up, it broke my heart. I just could not get it together. Too busy during the day to pump, did not drink enough water. I was probably not eating enough too, in retrospect.*
- *Give yourself a break, while we have all learned the physiologic and emotional benefits of breastfeeding for both moms and babies, know that your child will be happiest and healthiest when you are happiest and healthiest and if pumping is making you miserable, it's not worth it. You may be able to continue with just one or two feedings a day even if you can't pump throughout the day.*

Breastfeeding, bottle-feeding, and pumping are all pretty hot topics over at Mothers in Medicine. There are many posts with plenty of commentary that you may find helpful.

Childcare

Childcare is such a huge issue for working parents. It can be so expensive, and it is so important. With me in outpatient primary care and my husband traveling for his work pretty frequently, we needed to figure it out.

Usually, it's nanny vs. daycare. For some, a partner is willing and able to stay at home. For others, an unemployed, trustworthy, and enthusiastic family member is available. My mom is the reason we relocated before we had kids, and why hubby and I can pursue our careers. She is grandma/nanny/superhero. These days she picks up our kids from school and watches them at her house until one of us (usually me) can fetch them. She loves spending time with her grandkids, they adore her, and we pay her a small stipend. Win/win/win.

Family help is the best, but it can't always work, for many reasons. We have also used daycare, as well as nanny services, both to give my mom a break and to provide playmates for our kids.

Daycare has the advantage of providing key socialization, as well as building relationships with other working parents, a bonus that I didn't realize would be, until it was. However, if we didn't have my mom to pick up our kids at the end of the day, we'd be pretty miserable. It probably wouldn't work at all.

I found nannies to be the most difficult. It was almost a part-time job to find a decent nanny, even with helpful websites. And they weren't always decent. Plus, that option can be very expensive, prohibitively so.

Other docs have written about au pairs, and that option sounds wonderful, but one has to have a place for the person to sleep, and we just never had that. It's a small house, barely enough room for us and the two kids. Au pair, sadly, was never a possibility for us.

In the end, most folks will be examining the costs and benefits of a nanny or au pair situation against a home or freestanding daycare.

From families who chose daycare:

We chose daycare because we weren't too keen on a nanny or au pair. It's stressful to both hire a single person who is responsible for your child, and to have another person so close in your living space. Not for us. A good quality daycare facility provides good socialization with both adults and other children. However, the wrinkle is that as an anesthesiologist, my hours start well before any daycares that I have access to are open. My husband used to watch baby, prep for daycare and take her there in the morning, but sometimes he has to travel and it's a lot to do when trying to start work as well. So we hired an early morning "nanny-taxi" who watches baby for about 2 hours and then takes her to daycare each morning. It's working out well, but the only issue is that if there is something I want to communicate to the daycare about my child, it can be lost a bit in the translation when the nanny communicates it second-hand.

—*PracticeBalance*

I really didn't like the idea of being depending on one person for child care. I don't mind having my schedule upended when my kid gets sick. I didn't want to have my schedule upended when someone *else's* kid got sick. Eve started group day-care when she was about eight months old (we'd each been on part-time leave until then and we filled in the gaps with a family friend as sitter). She stayed there for preschool and then after school care through 4th grade.

—*Jay*

On Having an Au Pair

After doing daycare/preschool exclusively for a time (when we only had my daughter), a live-out nanny, and a live-in nanny at various times, we went the au pair route 1 1/2 years ago and couldn't be happier. It's just what our family needs right now. I wish I had known more about it earlier on, since it may have made life easier and richer back then. People may have had different experiences, but here's ours.

We've had two au pairs so far, and both turned out to be great matches for our family. The matching process reminds me a little of residency matching, but without the rank list. You search through au pair profiles, filtering by what's important to your particular family (maybe a strong driver or experience with taking care of multiple children or a particular religion), can read a "personal statement," watch a video they made to tell you more about themselves, scan their letters of recommendation, and their childcare experience. You can select au pairs to interview (via Skype generally) and have a certain amount of time to render a decision whether you want to match with the au pair. The au pair must accept the match as well, and you agree on an arrival date. It was a bit unnerving to select our au pairs, not knowing exactly how it would turn out in the end - would she like living with us? Would we like living with her? How would she be with the kids? Like residency matching, you go a lot by feel of a program and projected fit.

What we didn't anticipate was how much our au pairs would be like family to us. They have launched out on their own, excited to see the U.S. - everything is new. You are their host mom and dad, and it does feel a little like that - parental and guiding, showing them the ropes and helping them have a good experience in a new country. Our au pairs have been from Mexico and Brazil; we've learned about their countries. Last year, I made a Mexican Christmas dinner with our au pair at the time N; this year Brazilian.

N was with us for only 6 months. This is not typical. The contract is for a year. However, N's family needed her back home; a family member was ill so she had to break her end of the contract and our au pair company arranged for us to match with someone new. M, from Brazil, has been with us for almost a year. We love her. The kids love her. She loves being here. She's extended her contract for an additional year (the maximum possible) which is great news. There's a ramp up period of about a month when they first arrive for driving lessons, figuring out routines, roles, etc, so having her want to stay longer is a huge plus. Meanwhile, we keep in touch with N who writes me occasionally and updates me on her career and relationships. She's getting married next year and has invited our family to Mexico for it. It's kind of like a mentor/mentee relationship.

An au pair's hours have certain restrictions; they can provide a maximum of 45 hours per week. With our youngest in half-day preschool, this gives us a chance to have a date night each week or coverage on the occasional weekend day I have to work. She picks up the kids from school, drives them to their swim lessons, gets them bathed. We juggle the days and hours when there is an unexpected snow day or sick day. That flexibility has been key. You have to have space for an au pair to have his/her own room and be okay with someone living with you.

—KC, *"On having an au pair,"* December 19, 2013

Additional Commentary

I found Au Pair in America because my friend had used them and had a good experience. Cultural Care, Go Au Pair, and Au Pair Care are some others. Take a look at what the agencies say online about fees, rules, etc. It's definitely cheaper than a U.S. nanny, but there are more rules. What happens is you sign up (usually for a fee, but sometimes they waive it) and then you get permission to look at au pair profiles online. You also fill out some documents about your family so the au pair can see if she wants to work for you too. Then when you find an applicant you like, you send them an email and set up an interview over Skype. There are a couple of visits with a local coordinator as well. I think we started looking in November for a February placement, which was more than enough time. They recommend looking at least 2 months ahead of when you need one because it takes time to get their visa processed.

—OMDG, December 20, 2013

I think when it works well, it is amazing. I've heard horror stories too about feeling like you're the parent of an adolescent who stays out late partying etc. We've chosen women on the older range of 18-26, who have taken care of younger siblings etc. So far so good...

—K.C., Dec 21, 2013

What would be fantastic would be the normalization of quality, on-site daycare with doctor hours. Right now, this is an anomaly, something that a few of us have, but that many of us would love to have:

My hospital has a daycare that is open 6am to 8pm. Longer hours are key!

—Laura

I personally think this [onsite daycare with longer hours] is something we should all push for at every hospital. I have brought this up with the women physicians group at my institution as well, and they said they are working on it. So far, we have a new benefit of guaranteed backup care for 7 full days/year. But honestly, good quality daycare from 6 am to 8 pm should be a standard for every hospital that wants to hire physicians with families!

—PracticeBalance

[Onsite daycare with longer hours] is such a wonderful idea- It would boost productivity, no doubt. My colleagues who have to bolt out of here at 5:30 or 6 pm are stressed, unable to finish work, and then financially punished by the daycare if they are late!! Who does that help

—Genmedmom (me)

Working Mom Logistics (or, How to Create More Hours in the Day)

Let's face it: working moms have a lot on their plate. A patient recently complained to me how guilty she felt because she couldn't be a perfect mother, wife, accountant, and friend, all at the same time. If she felt strong in one area, she was slipping in another. "No matter how much I try, I'm a failure!" she declared.

Okay, look, despite the expectations on us, no one can achieve perfection 100% of the time. We are not going to excel in all of the areas of our lives always. But we can *manage*. We can do our myriad jobs *well enough*. And we can be *happy*.

On a weekly basis, I *usually* manage: four clinic sessions a week (approximately 20 hours seeing patients), one morning precepting in the first-year medical students' interviewing and communications course, co-parenting our two school-aged kids (with lots of family help), regular blogging on three separate blogs, kids' dinner/bathtime/bedtime virtually every night, about three good workouts per week, church and family dinner on Sundays.

Is it all done perfectly? Hell, no. I wish I could get to all the patient phone calls, emails, and lab results every week. It would be great if I could do the reading before the medical school course. Our kids are late with homework at least once per week. We never seem to know what's going on at school until the last minute. My blog posts often have typos and could use a little more editing. My workouts are sometimes *really* short. We don't get to church or have family dinner *every* Sunday.

But I can say this: We fit in what we need to fit in. We do what we feel needs to be done. It's not perfect, but, for us, it is. Imperfectly perfect. We, as a family, are happy.

I am often asked "Geez, how do you *do* it all?"

Well, if what you're aiming for is happiness rather than perfection, then I've thought about this. It will be different for everyone, but generally, I suggest:

Identify Your Time Wasters and Eliminate Them

What time-consuming things in your life *do not* help you to achieve your goals and *do not* serve a healthy purpose? For me, that's television. I do not watch television unless there is a really good reason. I'll watch a Disney movie with the kids once in a while, all snuggled on the couch. And, of course, once a week our whole family watches my husband's football team play. Other than that? No sitcoms, no news, no movies. Social media can also easily become a time-sucker, so I limit that to my train commute.

> We also hire help for activities that drain time and do not produce happiness, and I cannot stand the television, which brings so much time to my life.
>
> —Alyce, October 21, 2016

Hire Cleaners, If You Can

Yes, we all know that we are capable of cleaning. But how much is your time worth? As a physician, if you were paid by the hour, you would earn $100, at minimum. Multiply that by a thousand–no, a million–and that's how much your hour is worth to your kids. Though we couldn't afford it when we just started out, as soon as we could, we hired a cleaning service. They are worth every penny. And it doesn't hurt to have a very high tolerance for mess:

> I am highly tolerant of messes too, by necessity. It comes down to making choices… Are you going to spend the very little time you have, the precious irreplaceable time, with your kids baking, or making sure everything is neat? My five and three year old girls remember the projects we have done. They have yet to tell me-'Mommy you were so good to wipe the handle after I messed it all up with paint'.
>
> —Mommyhospitalist

Order Anything Online That Can Be Ordered Online

We have groceries, pet supplies, clothes, shoes, furniture, books, etc. delivered right to our front door.

Agree, ordering online (with speedy delivery) is the way to go. Another thing, don't sweat the small stuff. How's that for easier said than done, but important nonetheless. And know when to and when NOT to multitask. And even when beyond the infant/toddler years, it's still so important and oft-forgotten to get some (more) SLEEP.

—T is @kind4kids, November 6, 2016

Stay Local

Need to run an errand? Planning to meet friends for dinner? Wants to take the kids somewhere fun? If possible, avoid driving time, and support local businesses to boot. Maybe there's a grocery store farther away that's cheaper or has more selection. Is it worth the extra costs in gas and time? If there are good stores and restaurants in your community, why not give them your business? Little kids don't necessarily want or need to go to big-deal, special places, like the museum in the city. Even if you only go to the local park or playground, they'll be thrilled to be with you and have your full attention. My kids have been to the same rinky-dink wildlife rescue and seen the same skunk, owl, and deer countless times, but they love going there. Heck, they're thrilled to be in our own backyard, as long as I'm not looking at my damn phone, and actually playing with them!

Schedule Carefully

There are so many options for kids' activities around us. It would be very easy to slip into driving-everyone-all-over-the-place-for-this-or-that-thing. We were forced to hold back quite a bit, as our son with autism doesn't handle a busy schedule very well and doesn't do drop-off events at all. So, we have a music teacher who meets them in my mom's home after school one day a week. And we choose family activities like hikes, trips to the farmer's market, and scouting (Boy Scouts), rather than kids-only classes like dance and tae kwon do. We've realized that this quieter, easier, more familiar approach results in less hustle and bustle, and doubles as family time.

I hire help for after school and activities so I can get home and cook instead of running around in the car... Echo you big time on house cleaners and not over scheduling!! Gotta have some family dinner time not just running around every evening to sports events after you've already worked hard all day.

—Gizabeth Shyder

Identify Toxic Relationships and Avoid Them

Okay, I'm wandering into therapeutic territory here, but the truth is, people who make us feel bad are a real drain on our precious time and energy. Conflict and negativity are distracting. We can't be our best selves *now* if we're reliving an argument or rethinking that weird conversation from *yesterday*. If there's a person around who consistently brings conflict and negativity into my day, I avoid them as much as possible. Likewise, if there are good, psychologically solid people who support me and boost my mood, then hey, I want to spend more time with them.

Keep Reasonable Goals

Whatever your goals are, go for them! But remember that no one is perfect one hundred percent of the time. Striving for perfection can lead to perpetual stress and disappointment. Personally, I think that's kind of liberating. I'm not striving for crazy achievements in any area. I'd like to take good care of my patients, be a decent teacher for my students, raise emotionally well-adjusted kids, keep on writing until it goes somewhere, stay as healthy as possible, and be actively engaged in our community. Like I said, it's not perfect, but, for us, it is. Imperfectly perfect. We, as a family, are happy.

> *"Perfectly imperfect" has been my mantra too. So far we've limited activities (kids are just 2 and 4) and hope to keep it that way. I try to be conscious of what I am prioritizing - i.e. Feel good about getting the workout in, rather than focusing on what didn't get done.*
>
> —*N, November 10, 2016*

Sleep Deprivation (Because There Are Only 24 Hours in a Day)

As I write this, my kids are six and four years old. Am I still sleep deprived? Hell, yes! My son has had a cough that wakes him and then he cries out and sometimes needs his inhaler. My daughter still wakes up every third night or so and ends up in our bed. Then our cats think that we're awake to feed them and start knocking things off the bedside table. Anticipating all of this disturbance, you'd think that I would go to bed earlier, but let's face it, when I am flat-out exhausted, those few precious hours after the kids fall asleep are my only personal hours of the day. Hubby (if he's not traveling) and I divide and conquer the end-of-day tasks like dishes, kids' lunches, laundry, etc., then I catch up on the day's clinic work if needed, and then I do FUN things. I'm usually brain-dead by that time, but I will sometimes do online shopping or social media silliness, *just because I can.*

But when the kids were younger, the nights were even worse. I remember truly struggling to get through the day and almost falling asleep at the wheel on my commute from work. And I am not the only one. Generally, it's this: If the kids don't sleep through the night, mom doesn't sleep through the night. There are all sorts of different approaches to the perennial problem of children who cry in the night. Or demand to be fed. Or climb into bed with you. Or all of the above. In the end, as with just about everything, we all need to decide what works best for us as individuals and families.

Experiences, opinions, and advices on sleep issues abound, with people advocating from both ends of the sleep solution spectrum, from Cry It Out to Attachment Parenting, and everything in between:

From a pediatric surgeon : Just my five cents here: Do not (ever!) disturb a working system. My kids are lousy sleepers. From day one. No napping except if I hold them. So, no napping :). My gifted and very, very intense little daughter is six now, and she still does not sleep through the night most nights. But she is mature enough now to get herself back to sleep, get herself a drink, go to the loo and stuff. Doesn't need me anymore. I still wake up, hearing her, since I am probably a bit paranoid, I am waking up with every move of any of my kids. My four year old son is sleeping through most nights, but won't fall asleep alone. So, he falls asleep next to me, which I see as bonding time, not much bonding time during these madly busy days, so I figure it's a good thing. Daddy is carrying him to bed afterwards, that works really well. (He comes back every night, though, but he just crawls into bed and doesn't need me, so I count this as sleeping through the night - I guess it's all about definitions :)) Littlest: 14 month old and probably years before sleeping through the night. She wakes up often. I breastfeed her, so she sleeps next to me in her crib. If I feed her, she falls right back to sleep, if I don't - hell breaks loose. I need my sleep to function, I cannot be not concentrated standing in the O.R. So - no sleep training here. I cope with just giving everyone what they need. And - sometimes I am exhausted and think there must be an easier way. But mostly, that's when they are exceptional needy, and mostly, there is/was a reason for it. Like a major growth spurt, mentally or developmentally. Or (like last week) four teeth at once. I learned with time, that I just follow the flow, and do what works best for us. And - eventually, they won't need you anymore - and you'll loose sleep about that! I don't worry about any books or counselors or basically anybody anymore. They don't live my life. If night time is the only real quality time I spend with my babies - so be it."

—Trinity

My oldest was a terrible sleeper - we ended up doing co-sleeping with musical beds until he was 19 months old so that we could all get some sleep. We tried a lot of things, but what finally worked was leaving him in his crib, and then sitting next to him, occasionally patting and shushing. The first night he screamed for 2 hours, which was pretty much hell, but I was there, patting him, so at least I didn't feel like I abandoned him. The next night he screamed for about 45 minutes and then slept for 5 hours. The next night he slept for 7 hours straight. I had tried straight Cry-It-Out before, with similar results as you had. Actually I'm amazed we even had another kid after that experience (fortunately kid #2 has been a dream sleeper in comparison). I had read the No-Cry Sleep Solution, but nothing in there seemed to help, but I did find helpful information in The Sleep Lady's Good Night, Sleep Tight: Gentle Proven Solutions to Help Your Child Sleep Well and Wake Up Happy by Kim West. This was pretty helpful with getting him to sleep without having to nurse him or hold him until he completely fell asleep. It's so hard!

—Anne

We had a 2-hour bedtime routine--it was a literally song and dance as our kids made us sing about ten songs (Twinkle Twinkle, Somewhere Over the Rainbow, songs from Mary Poppins and Sound of Music etc. etc.) and read about ten books. They cried every time we said "last song" or "last book". Finally we stuck to our guns and limited it to two picture books and three songs. Yes there was crying in the beginning, but that stopped after we grew some spines.

—Myblog

You seem to have gotten through the Cry-It-Out much better than I did as an anguished, desperate resident who needed to start studying for her boards. I like the justifications you made that help me, 7 years down the road, feel better now about my decision back then. As I said before, I have a wonderfully healthy, happy, intelligent 7 year old who never brings up the fact that he was hoarse for a week at 8 months. I fully believe that children are so malleable and adjustable - there is little we can do short of neglect and abuse in this wonderfully developed society to hurt them as long as we are loving them. Whatever method we choose, as long as we do it lovingly they will survive.

—Gizabeth Shyder

I still reject the notion that cry it out is the only option. I sleep trained my 3 year old when he was 15 months old without it. I have talked to many mothers from other counties who have never heard of cry it out method. Just like it is unlikely that CIO will cause psychological damage, it is also unlikely that people who do not use this method have sleep deprived toddlers and parents. My mom friends and I are well rested, and our toddlers sleep just fine, despite not using this method. Every child and his/her parent(s) are different. We should all be respectful of each other's choices

—Buttonchops

My favorite phrases from all of the above sleep advice and the take-away here:

- "Whatever method we choose, as long as we do it lovingly they will survive."
- "Every child and his/her parent(s) are different. We should all be respectful of each other's choices."
- "I don't worry about any books or counselors or basically anybody anymore. They don't live my life. If night time is the only real quality time I spend with my babies - so be it."

On-Call

Call can be so hard. But call means something different to all of us in medicine. My "call" now only means answering pages from home. But even that can get hairy. As many times as I've been on call, I have no graceful coping strategy.

One time, just as Hubby and I were herding our two wound-up kids upstairs toward bath time, my pager went off. Hubby said he could handle things, and I went to the dining room to call the patient.

It sounded like a simple upper respiratory infection that had triggered an asthma exacerbation, but I was asking a lot of questions to make sure it wasn't a really bad asthma attack and that there wasn't a high likelihood of pneumonia or some comorbidity to prompt urgent care.

Then: "What are you doing, Mommy?" My daughter wandered into the room.

Hubby was right behind her: "Come here, come back! Mommy has to make this phone call!"

"Who are you talking to, Mommy? Can I sit on your lap?" She started climbing up into my lap.

Meantime, I'm trying to continue: "Have you had any high fevers or chills?"

"MOMMY! Can I talk on the phone too? Can I have the phone?"

Then, my son ran into the room. "What is everybody doing? HEY get away from my Legos! Those are mine!" A tussle ensued. On my lap.

Screeching and wailing, grabbing, flailing, and some hitting.

Me, to the patient: "I am so sorry, please excuse the chaos over here…"

She, chuckling: "I raised four of my own. It's no problem at all."

We wrapped it up with a plan, and I hung up. She had all the medications she needed at home, so I didn't need to then also call in a bunch of prescriptions as well, thank goodness!

In the end, we all need to decide: Can I do this? Can I make this work? And if so, how am I going to cope?

Below, a post by an OB/GYN giving the surgeon on-call perspective and tips:

My Life As a Call Girl

I spend 1/4 of my life on call. With 10 years of private practice in OB/GYN under my belt that's 2.5 years that I've been tied to my phone. Some nights I sleep peacefully through the night, but more often than not, I get to trek in at 3 am to catch a baby or two. Over the years, I've come up with my own set of on call rules to help navigate the chaos that can be a call night.

Don'ts:

Don't dread it. *Obviously, I don't wake up on my call day with a spring in my step, open the windows and shout for joy for all to hear "Yeah, I get to be on call today!" But I don't dread it either. I've learned to deal with it and enjoy it the best I can. If I didn't make peace with being on call then, I end up wishing away a quarter of my life.*

Don't complain about it. *When I chose OB/GYN I chose a crazy, sleep deprived life. Sometimes when I'm working post-call I will "explain" to people why I look hot mess of disheveled craziness (i.e. I delivered 17 babies last night). I try to keep it in a upbeat joking tone and not a "Woe is me! I work all the time" tone. We all know those providers who claim that every single call is the "Worst call ever" and that is simply annoying.*

Don't indulge in the 3 am donuts. *When you are up all night, the 3 am donuts can look so very tempting. Sometimes I delude myself into thinking "I deserve a treat" for having to work all night, however my 40 year old metabolism does not agree and I regret it later. I always keep healthier snacks like almonds and trail mix with me for just such emergencies.*

Don't schedule appointments. *After getting called in half way through a haircut once, I learned this lesson the hard way.*

Don't socialize. *If my leaving the event will be awkward, I won't schedule it when I'm on call; like dinner with just one other couple. If it's a bigger group of friends, I will sometimes try to go if I can. Also having people over is definitely out as well. Having to rush out half way through cooking dinner is not a great plan.*

(continued)

Do's

Do live your life. *I can't put my life on hold completely when I'm on call. I still go to soccer games and church, I just drive separately in case I get called in. I still exercise, I just make sure when I'm running I have my phone on me and am always less than 10 min from my house. Sure this means that occasionally I have to race into the hospital all sweaty and get amniotic fluid on my Lulu tights but there are enough excuses not to exercise and I won't let call be one of them.*

Do keep some entertainment close by. *A lot of call can be "hurry up and wait." I often spend time waiting for an OR to open up or waiting for patient to deliver. I use this time for catch up charting and CME and reading. This is actually my one bit of call superstition: I always keep a novel with me in hopes I won't need it.*

Do Bathe. *My biggest pet peeve is getting called to the hospital stat when I'm in the middle of a shower. Yes, the ruptured ectopic pregnancy is far more important than me having a bad hair day, but still it's annoying. I wish I could get away with not bathing on call but that would not be socially acceptable. Instead, I keep extra toiletries handy to throw in the bag at the last minute as needed to get ready at the hospital.*

Do know your limits. *I am human. Occasionally, I need to ask for help. If a call is particularly awful I will get one my NPs to field phone calls. There are times I've cancelled part of my afternoon post-call to go home and rest. So no, I don't complain about every single call, but when I'm dangerously tired I listen to my body and rest.*

—RH+, "My Life as a Call Girl," May 26, 2015.

Let's Talk About Sexism

Let's talk about sexism. Seriously: mothers in medicine get an extra dose of this in pregnancy, nursing, and motherhood. The expectations for women in the workplace are ridiculous: If they are smart, they also need to be humble; strong, but also deferential; confident, but also really sweet; attractive, but not sexy…. It's too much.

Let's face it, for many folks, still, a "real" doctor looks like Marcus Welby, MD. You know, a white, gray-haired, suited man who exudes experience and wisdom. Not that there's anything wrong with that… Negative attitudes can manifest differently and span a wide range of experiences.

The way I see it, assumptions can be innocent. These can be sort of insulting things said by well-intentioned people. They may be based in inherent bias and unconscious attitudes. Like, for example…

How many times during residency training did I walk into a patient's room, and they assumed I was anyone but the doctor? I was asked to clear the cafeteria tray more than once. Even after introducing myself, I was often referred to as (insert non-physician staff title here) and asked to fetch things: a glass of water, blankets, a urinal.

Sometimes, those assumptions annoyed me, and I acted annoyed. Other times, I tried to be cheerful and helpful regardless. After all, I have also been guilty of making assumptions about others and have had to retrieve my Dansko-clad foot from my mouth.

What I observed throughout all of my medical training was that women received very little understanding, consideration, or flexibility during pregnancy, maternity leave, or breastfeeding. The prevailing attitude was "suck it up, buttercup." A woman I trained with had a miscarriage, and the supervising physicians would not allow her any time off. It was a first trimester loss. "Think of it like a heavy period," they said. "Would you call out for that?"

All of those crappy experiences and observations strengthened my resolve to work in a place that was as supportive as possible. And so, in that job search almost 10 years ago, I sought out a flexible position in a positive environment at a progressive institution, and I found it. The few negative experiences I had prior definitely informed my decision and helped me to recognize what I *didn't* want as an attending.

Here is what other doc-moms have encountered and what they feel about it:

I think the more appropriate question is: How have I NOT encountered sexism/discrimination in the workplace. It is implicit, cultural, ubiquitous. One of my laziest male resident counterparts quipped about my maternity leave: "So nice you are getting extra vacation." No. While you were on vacation, I was saving mine for the hardest, most important job of my life. That's one example of many, but it does us no good to stay bitter. I think this is changing, although the current political climate seems to belie that. Pushing progress means not being satisfied with settling in the norm. We have to break out of our cultural expectations. Push the envelope. March, do, and act for the future, for our children.

—*Gizabeth Shyder, January 13, 2017*

Yes, I am also from the Northeast and have gotten feedback which boils down to, essentially, smile more. I am an even keeled person but not much of an extrovert, and I work in a setting where we deal with some pretty heavy issues. Yet, I feel like I have to walk around all day with a giant smile plastered on my face at all times or I'm going to get in trouble. Meanwhile, the male physicians can even snap at people or be short, never mind not smiling, and it's just shrugged off.

—*Dad3mass, January 13, 2017*

As I tell my friends, a female physician has to be so much better than their male counterparts to be heard and respected because society is only starting to appreciate our communication styles, our voices, and our hard work to keep it together.

I've had to play the quiet and sweet intern because the nurses would call the "mean" interns for ridiculous issues in the middle of the night, i.e. Enema order. When I told my male attending this story, he said he's yelled at them for this. The male interns who are decent or cute get the female staff to bend to their will and don't give them any protests when they're rude. I think part of the problem is women not supporting other women.

Being an attending now, I make an effort to talk about the balance as a mother and a physician to our male and female residents. The more they hear, I hope they understand and can be supportive of another. I've told them if they have an issue with the culture or have a family issue, that family comes first and as co-workers we need to support that. Burn out is real when we don't feel supported.

—*g.t,. January 22, 2017*

Specialty Considerations

As an internist, it's hard for me to imagine what other specialist-moms experience. Some specialities are hard to imagine, if you're not in it. So, why not let them tell us? Below, essays from a medical researcher and a neurosurgeon:

Medical Research: Chasing Funding

By Sarita Patil, MD, Instructor in Allergy and Immunology

The very nature of biomedical research can make balancing career duties and family difficult. Our current research infrastructure in most US institutions requires a constant pursuit of funding. To complicate matters, most physician-scientists exist on "soft money" in the sense that the research position, let alone the research, is funded by grants and revenue brought into the lab, rather than a stipend or another more dedicated revenue stream. So while most fellows in training have protected research time to pursue their researchers, after the transition to a young investigator, the need to "protect" one's research time becomes critical.

For physician-scientists as well as clinical researchers, the balance of research duties, whether at the wet bench, with patients, or doing data analysis, requires space and time. For physician-scientists who work at the bench, finding dedicated time to carry out experiments that often don't fit within the typical 8-5 work day and balancing those with your family's needs can be difficult. Most mothers, like myself, have often worked after children are asleep or before they start their day to carve out the necessary time. Sustaining this over long periods of time is challenging, and most young investigators find that they need experimental support in the form of technical assistance to propagate their research careers. For clinical studies, coverage for the studies often extends before the 8-5 time span, and often has to be carefully negotiated with both coworkers and one's spouse.

Finding the technical assistance and support from research infrastructure can also be challenging at this career stage. As one's career grows, and additional personnel are hired, again the need to continue to pursue sustained funding for the research as well as hired personnel, who we often also mentor, becomes paramount. One other critical aspect of a research career is support from the department and administrative level, which is essential for career support and development.

Advice that I've gotten previously is that the single most important element of embarking on a research career is to find a mentor. For physician-scientist mothers, having a supportive mentor is critical. Life is complicated, and children/partners/yourself become ill and need you. At those times, it's critical to have a mentor who is accepting and supportive of your efforts. It can be hard to gauge these characteristics ahead of time, but I think it helps to have mentors who are themselves active participants in their family lives and who are sympathetic to the human condition.

As one of my strong female mentors has told me, it also helps to have a very thick skin. The research world in general is not always friendly to mothers, and the thick skin has been helpful. This particular mentor is a phenomenal example of a strong female role model. She is a senior physician scientist at an elite institution who believes so strongly in mentorship that she literally told me that she would continue to mentor me after I left her institution—and she has been my rock every since then. She has never hesitated to give brutally frank advice about the big things and very practical nuggets about the smaller ones. Everyone should be so fortunate to have someone like her.

As for my path in research, there have been a few critical elements. I chose a young, energetic mentor who is strongly supportive of me and my family life. (A side note here: He had a family while going through medical school and subsequent training which may have made him more sympathetic but I suspect the real factor is that he is a truly stellar human being.) He also recognized the need for female mentorship and has actively encourage female mentorship for me, even cross-institution. My partner in life is also supportive of my research career, having had been an academic himself previously. Finally, my family has been very supportive, with my mother literally helping me with the overnight care of my child, so that I could write a grant to fund and sustain my career during my maternity leave. My family has also come in to pinch hit when I have frequent travel or when we have emergency illnesses. I am also fortunate to be surrounded by mother physician-scientist mothers, at my institution who support and encourage each other.

It's Not Rocket Science...

...but it is brain surgery! Neurosurgery has always seemed to have a certain aura and mystique about it as a specialty. It certainly was glamorous to me when I started out as a medical student. After all, neurosurgeons work in and around the **brain***, the seat of our very existence. In fact, we work more often on the spine than the brain, but nonetheless, we are "brain surgeons."*

I was one of those annoying medical school classmates who started from Day 1 wanting to do neurosurgery, and who continued that path relentlessly, without second thoughts. Having walked the long and difficult road, I will say unequivocally that it is in NO WAY family friendly. It's hard to think of a less family friendly specialty. That's one reason why, even today, only 5% of about 3500 practicing neurosurgeons in the US are women.

There are oodles, scads, of reasons why this is the case.

1. Long and difficult training: Residency is an average of 7 years duration (usually not counting fellowship). Even so, it is hard to learn everything you need to know: patient evaluation, types of pathology, technical skills, reading your own radiographic studies, etc. The days are long and exhausting. I don't know how it is now, since the 80 hour work week, but I suspect it's still very demanding. It's difficult to carve out time and energy for your family. It's also hard to be pregnant during residency, the prime child bearing years.

2. Lots of emergencies: Problems like acute brain hemorrhages and cauda equina syndromes can't wait. In fact, sometimes half an hour makes all the difference. This makes planning your day impossible. As soon as you make plans to go out to the theater with your husband or go to your son's football game, the surgery gods conjure up a subdural. Curse you, surgery gods!

3. Unsympathetic colleagues: This specialty is full of men with stay at home wives who do everything for them. Nothing against SAHM's!! But don't expect your fellow residents or partners to understand taking breaks for breastfeeding. Don't expect them to help you in any way, because they have NO IDEA what your life is like outside work.

4. All or none: There is no such thing as a part time neurosurgeon. Trust me, I've seen it tried.

5. Physically demanding: This specialty demands long hours standing without a break. The sleep deprivation and stress are extremely taxing. Even after residency, there are times when you are so tired that you can't decide whether to eat or sleep first. This is after 24+ hours without a proper meal. Sex? Sleep is better when you haven't slept for 2 days! Add a crying baby to the nights you are home...

6. Culture: In neurosurgery, asking for any help is a sign of weakness. Call me if you need me... but don't call me. This culture is not conducive to supporting things like maternity leave.

7. Help wanted: Out in practice, when most of us are rearing teenagers, it would be great to have lots of partners to share call and PAs to help with the workload. Good luck with that. There is a chronic shortage of neurosurgeons; the ones that exist are difficult to recruit. It took us 4 years to find one to replace a partner who left. PAs are in high demand and would much rather take cushy dermatology jobs than difficult neurosurgical ones. I currently take call every 4th night and consider myself lucky.

8. Social isolation: I didn't expect this to be such a problem. Nonetheless, it has a large effect on our social life as a family. We don't get invited places because friends think I'm too busy. (Or maybe they just secretly don't like me, but this is what they tell me!) At church and school functions, people don't chat with us, they ask me about their aunt's brain tumor treatment. Even neurosurgeons like to talk about the weather and the upcoming football game, y'all!

So having said all that, you may well ask: "Why would anyone ever want to do this awful job?!"

(continued)

There are oodles of reasons for that, too.

1. It's surgery! How could anyone not love doing surgery? I've said it before... fixing a problem by opening the body and closing it again, and having the patient survive the experience, is nothing short of a miracle to me. It still amazes me after 10 years of practice.

2. Control: As an extreme Type A, I love controlling everything about what I do. I own my practice with my partners, so I am my own boss. What I say in the OR and in the office, goes. My own decisions and actions determine my patients' outcomes, and that's the way I want it.

3. Impact: Every day, I see patients with life-threatening problems. Through my profession, I am able to save lives and keep people out of wheelchairs. Being able to make a real difference in just one person's life makes it all worthwhile. In neurosurgery, that impact on the patient is so often immediate and dramatic. It's high risk, but high reward.

4. Respect: This specialty still commands immense respect, both from patients and colleagues. Not that we deserve more respect than other professions, but there it is.

5. Financial security: It's still a good living, although politics may change that in years to come. Not having to always worry about money is one less strain on a marriage. Further, a neurosurgeon can always provide for herself and her kids should that become necessary.

6. The Challenge: This may be the thing I love most about my job. Every day, every patient, every case brings a new challenge. There are always new things to learn, envelopes to push. I never get bored or complacent, because it's just not possible. Towards the end of residency, I once thought I'd seen it all. Later that day, the nurse at the trauma desk popped her head up to ask, "Hey, are you seeing the guy that got assaulted by the ostrich?!" Never a dull moment!

I love neurosurgery and can't imagine doing anything else. Family friendly? Nooooo. Worth it? Yes! It can be done, although it's not easy. As others here have pointed out, no working mom has an easy time of it. All we can do as MiM's is give it our best and hope that the ones we love understand us and continue to love us back.

—*GCS15, "It's not rocket science!" December 16, 2011.*

Summary and Conclusions

I hope that the take-home message here has been loud and clear: Take all the advice with a big grain of salt, and do whatever is right for you and your family. The ideas and suggestions here are merely intended to provide illustration, as well as reassurance and validation! From here, go and do what you think will work for your situation. And then, share it with the rest of us at Mothers in Medicine. Because that's what we as doctors, mothers, and mentors need to do: Support each other. It's a special community and we welcome your input.

References

1. Keen RR, et al. Occupational hazards to the pregnant orthopaedic surgeon. J Bone Joint Surg Am. 2011;93:e141(1-5).
2. Fowler JR, Culpepper L. Working during pregnancy. UpToDate. 2015.
3. The Centers for Disease Control, Emergency Preparedness and Response. Radiation and Pregnancy: A Fact Sheet for Clinicians. http://emergency.cdc.gov/radiation/prenatalphysician.asp.

Chapter 5
Choosing Where and How to Work

Andrea Flory

I got married near the end of my last year of residency. When I started medical school, in fact when I started residency, I hadn't yet even met my husband, and I didn't have any of the 3 kids I now have. That's probably a good thing because I would surely have talked myself out of the specialty I really loved into something more "family-friendly". There's nothing wrong with family-friendly, mind you. I always read the classified ads in the New England Journal just out of curiosity, wondering whether there are more part-time jobs cropping up as women, who more often work part-time than men in general, represent a greater share of young doctors. So far, I don't think much has changed in the job advertising sphere.

When I happen to have a bad day at work, which is fortunately rare, I permit myself to back up and take a different fork in the road. In my alternate life, maybe I became a dermatologist, where "full-time" seems to be 4 days a week…but who works full-time anyway? Or infectious diseases, where every other ad seems to start "Full-time or part-time". Ah, travel clinic…seeing some healthy people and getting them ready to travel to exotic locales. Lest fear of boredom be a factor, keep in mind that the occasional traveler will come home with a fever of 40.8—is it malaria? Dengue fever? Ebola? See, that would spice things up. And clinic finishes at 3p.

But snap out of it. I became a medical oncologist, had my first baby midway through my second year of fellowship, another baby at the end of my third year, and a third baby about a year and a half into my first "real job". At some point in late second year when other fellows were beginning to do their job talks and interviews, it dawned on me that I didn't want to be away from my son and his future sibs for 60 hours a week. I didn't want to miss first steps or first words or first anythings. It didn't feel right to me that someone other than me—indeed, someone I hadn't even met yet—would be there for more of my kids' waking hours than I would, and that's exactly what working full-time meant.

—Tempeh, "How to get a part-time job in medicine," November 18, 2008

The original version of this chapter was revised. An erratum to this chapter can be found at https://doi.org/10.1007/978-3-319-68028-6_12

A. Flory, MD (✉)
Washington, DC, USA
e-mail: alflory@gmail.com

As a child, it was always clear to me that my life was intended for meaningful work. After all, I was the tallest girl in my class; I knew that was a sign of my responsibility. Everyone told me I was smart. My social worker mother and nurse grandmothers showed me that women could care for people outside as well as inside the home. My family culture and community church told me that helping others was the highest good a person could do.

In addition, I could see for myself that other people needed help. I noticed the disheveled man rummaging through the sidewalk trash can for food as I held my mother's hand. Later, my surprised parents wondered how my 8-year-old self was planning to get to the home of the blind church members to whom I had apparently volunteered to read. As I grew older, the earnest and philosophical young adult novels I favored told me the same thing—there was work to be done, and we owed the world our best effort. I considered training as a nurse, like my grandmothers or the ones in the Cherry Ames books. Then a beloved family friend, just home from delivering her son, proclaimed "There are lots of great nurses, but we need more female doctors," and I heard my calling.

In medical school, primary care spoke to me. I loved the detective work of investigating a brand-new symptom and was impressed by the power of the trust between a patient and his physician. I felt the pressure to pick a specialty with more glamour or income, but primary care felt like the essence of helping to me.

When I finished residency in Providence, I was excited to get out of the hospital and finally practice in the real world. I was happily dating where I was, so rather than move back to DC as planned, I took a job in a multi-specialty community practice in a nearby small town. The female physician who led the practice was someone I knew and admired. She was tough but fair. Everyone in the practice was expected to work hard, but there was a great sense of community with the patients who came to see us. Even the police officer who pulled me over for expired plates recognized me from the walk-in clinic; he apologized for having to tow my car and then drove me to work in his patrol car!

As a young attending, my work filled my days. My helpfulness and attention to detail endeared me to my patients and I adored them back. I didn't mind the way my clinic spilled into lunch and my charts filled my weekday evenings. I still managed a social life, enjoyed my hobbies and exercise, and had plenty of time for long baths and leisurely meals. I spent too much time worrying I would never have the family I wanted but was generally satisfied being the doctor I had dreamed of becoming.

Eventually, I tired of being a single woman in a town that seemed to be filled with extended families. All my close friends had spouses and young families; I was sick of tagging along. I wanted to be comfortable going to a movie or a restaurant alone, which never felt normal in Providence. I missed the diversity and variety of DC life. I hoped that I would have better luck in finding a partner with whom I could build my own family there. So, I moved back.

By the time I married, in my mid-30s, I was working for my old medical school, doing adult primary care and teaching students. It was engrossing work but harder in some ways than my previous job. The clinic was fast-paced and sometimes chaotic. My patients were sicker and had more barriers to care—and it took longer to earn their trust. Teaching medical students was intimidating at first, but I soon found my groove and loved it.

Fortunately, my husband also had a job with crazy hours. We made our marriage work by having independent workdays and restricting our time together to the weekends. By the time we started seriously contemplating having a child, neither of us could imagine how we could add a kid to the mix. I wasn't sure anymore that it was a good idea. For one thing, so many things could go wrong with a late pregnancy, and I suspected that it would be my hard-earned career that would suffer if we had to care for a child with a chronic illness. While I loved my husband very much, the union of two strong-willed, independent people did not make for the easiest of marriages; I worried that adding the stress of a child might compromise our relationship.

My husband felt otherwise. He was certain that a child would enrich our lives. I decided to squelch my uncertainty and to trust him. We started to make changes to make space for a baby: he moved from his consuming law firm job to a lower-paying government position, and I arranged to work 4 days per week. My pregnancy was easy enough and I worked up to my due date. After our son was born, I chose to stay home with him for four largely-unpaid months. While I loved spending time with him, I felt restless at home. We found a wonderful caregiver, and I went back to work.

Shortly after my son's first birthday, my responsibilities at work increased significantly. I was offered a medical school role that encompassed both the leadership of a large, established course and a rapid revision of that subject area to update and integrate it into a reworking of the overall medical student curriculum. There was no question that I wanted the position. While I recognized that it would be a tremendous amount of work, it was a topic about which I felt passionate. I was confident I could make positive changes and was excited to have the power to influence medical students in how they would care for future patients. My clinical work was reduced to allow for additional teaching and administrative time. We made plans to shift tasks around at home to account for my increased time at work. My husband and I expected that the first year or so would be rough, but then things would settle into a more regular routine.

That first year was incredibly difficult: intimidating, exciting, and exhausting. I felt unmoored, unsure of my decisions and frazzled by the amount of choices and plans that had to be made quickly. My advisors and helpers were also pulled in a thousand directions, so I learned to work efficiently and stopped second-guessing my decisons. As the months went on, the work continued to pile up. With un-meetable responsibilities in my clinical practice, medical school roles, and at home, I triaged remorselessly. Someone was always being shortchanged, but I tried to manage my guilt by rotating which areas got my attention.

As the first year stretched into two years and then three, it became harder and harder to maintain the pace. It was clear that more hands were needed but help was slow to arrive. There were signs of burnout; I dreaded going to work, was less efficient when I was there, and felt strung out much of the time. At home, I worked frantically to keep up with housework and chores—everything was done in a rush. I would calculate how much time I had to make a pot of soup before the dryer finished or plot how to combine errands to complete them in a single trip. My husband was frustrated that I was still so consumed by work, and my son, now 4, craved all my attention when I was home. I worried that I was missing too much of his life.

Beyond the tensions at work and home, I began to resent the loss of my personal time. Yes, my work felt important and was fulfilling, but I missed my friends. I missed entertaining, traveling, reading novels, having long conversations, and being outdoors. All of those had been given away in exchange for my work.

Looking back, it seems clear that I should have been thinking seriously about finding another job. At the time, however, it was not as obvious. Surrounded by a group of people who keep long hours and make sacrifices for work, doing a job I considered worthwhile, and lacking someone to whom I could hand off my project, I did not have the wherewithal to see it. I could not imagine trying to look for a new job. It was not until my husband emailed me a detailed financial plan for my unemployment that it occurred to me that I could simply leave my job. It was an amazing idea to me. Shortly thereafter, I submitted a letter of resignation.

It has been almost 2 months since I left my work and I am relishing the slower pace of my unemployment. I am still recovering; it has taken time to recalibrate. I continue to teach a bit, but most of my time is spent catching up on the things I have missed: time with my family, sleep, neglected house chores, and connecting with friends. I am so grateful to have this time.

I have started to ruminate a bit about future work and my thoughts center on the most basic of branch points. What role do I want my work to play at this point in my life? It seems to me that there are two possible paths to consider. I can choose to look for a new leadership role—what I think of as "important work" or "a big job," the kind of work that will stretch and challenge me in new ways—or I could choose a clinical primary care job, difficult in its own way, but relatively comfortable after 15 years of practice.

Of course, it is a false choice. There are intermediate shades in between those two and many combinations that might work. The conundrum lies in the philosophical underpinning. If I pick an "easy" job, am I doing enough? Am I helping enough people, working hard enough, fulfilling my feminist leadership responsibilities enough? Alternatively, if I choose a "big" job, am I sacrificing my family or my happiness to my own need for a sense of purpose? How do I chart my new course?

One of the privileges of my work, both as a primary care physician and as an educator, has been the chance to hear people's stories and the intimate details of their lives. I have observed how people make choices, both big and small. The most important thing I have learned is that decisions are extremely personal and that every option in a difficult choice has aspects that will be both positive and negative for that individual. With rare exceptions, there is no universal right choice. Given that, how can you make the best career and family choices?

Making the Best Balanced Work/Life Choices

Take Away the Pressure to Find the one Perfect Specialty or Job

Whatever you choose will probably work out well in some ways and less well in others. It will have downstream consequences that you should consider but will not be able to predict completely. Each choice opens some doors and closes others, at least temporarily.

Know Yourself Well

Unflinching self-knowledge can help you choose a life that gives you purpose and sustains you while minimizing the things that are likely to tire and frustrate you. In choosing medicine, we all committed to a life of service. It seems a simpler choice, however, when we are only giving our own time and energy. Things become more complicated when our own work choices compromise the ability to care for and enjoy our families. The second shift of parenthood limits the opportunities for self-care and recovery from work, so the personal cost of work is amplified. In addition, motherhood can change our values and perspectives. Caring for the vulnerable may carry more weight, demonstrating a life true to personal ethics may become more critical, and we may recognize more acutely how the choices we make play out over an extended time. Parenting also expands our skill set; those same clever tricks that get a toddler to eat can be repurposed on a reluctant administrator who does not like the options in front of him.

We commonly talk about work/life balance, leaning in and having it all, but those ideas get tricky in application. Our time and energy are limited resources, so while efficiency and smart planning can help maximize them, we had better make sure that the most critical needs and desires get priority. Every year in medical school orientation, one of our deans tells the story of the professor who fills a jar with rocks, pebbles, and sand. If you put all the sand in first, she explains, it fills the jar with small things and there is no room for the larger rocks. But if the largest rocks go in first, then there is room for the pebbles and the sand in the space they leave behind. If we can determine our priorities and place them first in our lives, then the smaller needs and wants can fit in the space around them.

Figure out what is most important to you. For a medical student considering specialty choices: which rotations did you enjoy most and, more importantly, what about them did you love? Was it pondering the mystery of an unknown diagnosis or the satisfaction of fixing something with your own hands? Do you want the surety of mastering everything about your subspecialty or the excitement of not knowing what might show up next? Think about your interests and hobbies outside of medicine; sometimes they can help you make the connection to what is most vital. Given that all careers have both joy and hassle, what do you imagine would be the best parts of a job for you? For trainees and career-changers: consider the aspects of your current (or most recent) position that were best. What did you love doing? What connects you to the reasons you entered medicine? If you are making a change, what did not work? How do you want things to be different for you?

Don't judge your own preferences or values. It is dangerous to invest years of energy and time training in a specialty because you think it will be best for family life, if you do not love the work. Similarly, your grandmother may have held her obstetrician in highest esteem, but if you get queasy in the OR and are miserable when you are up all night, it will be hard for you to enjoy that work, no matter how much you would like to please her. Accept what is most important to you and your choices will be much easier to live with.

Recognize your personal biases and how they influence your ideas about what is acceptable. Many of us carry invisible boundaries that we learned early in life that may make certain choices seem transgressive. For example, it may not feel right for your husband to go part time to care for your baby, while you go back to work full time, even if you consider yourself an ardent feminist, because it conflicts with your unconscious expectations of how a man or a mother "should" behave. Making the biases conscious allows you to decide whether they are true and if they apply to your current situation.

Similarly, pay attention to the personal narratives that you tell yourself. We often make up our mental autobiographies based on a fallible interpretation of our life events and how we think other people perceive us. They may also contain echoes of things that we heard as children, like "Jenny is too lazy to be a leader" or "Sara needs to learn to keep her mouth shut." If we do not hear those stories for what they are, they can have an undeserved power to become our self-image and to influence our choices.

Make Choices Consistent with your Values

Define a personal and/or family "mission statement." This is a succinct summary of the values and desires that you wish to embody as a person or family. Creating one forces you to decide what is most important to you as a person or family (the rocks in the analogy above). You may want to make one specific to your career as well, which can describe your professional focus. Once you have a mission statement, use it as a tool to help choose which specialty or job option is most consistent with your priorities. It can also help you give yourself permission to say no when offered a role that is not consistent with your vision.

Make choices with a clear head whenever possible. Be ready with phrases that allow you to politely refuse to make an immediate decision, e.g., "That sounds like a great offer. Give me the weekend to think about it and I will get back to you on Monday." Avoid making a choice when you are tired or upset. Get some real or psychological space from your current situation before making a change. Do use friends or mentors as advisors, but be aware of how their own interests or biases may affect their opinions about your decisions. Be cautious when revealing information to those who may have conflicts of interest.

Gather practical information about your options. Be realistic about the commitment that new career or social roles are likely to require of you. When looking at a new job, get as much information as you can about things like typical work hours, time required outside of work, and travel requirements. Try to get a sense of expectations that leadership may have for research, meetings, teaching, or administrative work that is not spelled out in a job description or contract.

Consider going part time. Part time can be a great choice when you have a growing family, since it allows you both professional satisfaction and more time to spend with family and get things done at home. If you do choose part-time work, be sure that you understand how it changes your pay and benefits, which can decrease more than proportionally. In addition, you may find that call and other expectations may not be lightened much when you decrease time at work. You will want to be sure that you will have appropriate coverage for all professional roles when you are out of the office. Decreasing from full-time work also has the potential to affect your advancement in academic or organizational settings.

Other creative options may exist, depending on your area of specialty and location. You may be able to telework or complete some work at home. You may be able to swap some clinical time for additional academic or administrative responsibilities, which tend to be more flexible. Alternatively, there may be walk-in clinic, hospital work, or nonclinical jobs in industry or the government that may offer more manageable hours for those who want to cut back.

Know your value. Understand how much leverage you are likely to have in a particular negotiation and use it to get what you need most. Remember that negotiation can be tricky for women; we can be penalized both for asking and for not asking for raises or promotions, so learn the best ways to engage. Consider your employer's position, and see if you can find a way to frame your request that acknowledges those interests. You may want to practice role-playing the conversation, especially if you anticipate a challenging interaction.

Honor your intuition if something does not seem right when you are exploring a new position. There is no extra credit given for putting yourself in a punishing situation or tying yourself to someone who does not have your best interests at heart. Both medical training and attending jobs can be difficult to leave because of contract requirements, responsibilities to patients, and other factors, so make sure that you have the information you need before accepting an offer.

Lastly, be Ready to Course-Correct if Needed

What if you pick the wrong specialty, choose a bad job, or find that your priorities have changed? You cannot always anticipate what the consequences of a choice will be. When that happens, be truthful in looking at your thinking and motivations. Figure out what you can learn from the situation, review your priorities, and decide your next move.

As for me, I have no regrets about my choices so far. I feel lucky to have done work that I chose and was meaningful to me. I am thankful to have my family and the pause in my career to enjoy them. The next step is a mystery, but I am excited to see what waits in store.

Chapter 6
Balancing Work and Life

Jenni Levy

> *Anyone else ever get so busy and stressed out that they start imagining how awesome it would be to have appendicitis?*
>
> —RH+, *Stressed Out, October 7, 2012*

She wasn't the only one. Twelve commenters agreed with her, and I've had my days of envying my patients who got to *lie in bed and watch TV!* I've been a doc since 1986 and became a mom in 2000. I've worked in hospitals and outpatient primary care offices and been a hospice medical director and done palliative care consults and taught residents and medical students. I've worked part-time and full-time and I've stayed home, at least briefly. None of those incarnations allowed me to stay in bed and watch TV—and, to be honest, I'd probably hate it after the first two hours.

I'm supposed to write about balance—that mythical Eden where we can have it all—the work we love, the family we cherish, the "me time" everyone says we need, and enough sleep. Ah, enough sleep. Sigh. Work-life balance is a hot topic for all women, although as long as we frame this as a "women's issue," we will not be able to build societal solutions for the problems that men and women face. If women are talking about balance, women in medicine—especially mothers in medicine—will certainly be talking about it, agonizing about it, wishing for it, and writing about it. We've had two topic weeks on work-life balance, one in 2008 and the other in 2010. Our regular bloggers and several guests, as well as our wonderful commenters, wrote about the precariousness of their lives and the way they made things work— or didn't:

J. Levy, MD, FAACH (✉)
Jenni Levy, LLC, Allentown, PA, USA
e-mail: advanceplanningpa.com

© Springer International Publishing AG 2018
K. Chretien (ed.), *Mothers in Medicine*,
https://doi.org/10.1007/978-3-319-68028-6_6

Hubby and I barely see each other – this month I'm working nights in Emergency and he's on 1:4 call for the general surgery service. I think we spent less than 8 hours awake in each other's company this week. I never seem to have time to study or read around cases. Hubby feels like he's barely prepared for days in the OR and for exams. I feel like I could be a better doctor if only there was more time or energy. And this beautiful child, well, he doesn't like to sleep much. And although my brain screams "No Way!", my heart is ready for another baby (or two). How do you other Mothers in Medicine make it work?

—Anonymous, "Resident Mom Barely Keeping Head Above Water", December 15, 2010

Fizzy explained how she managed as a resident with a baby: she stayed out of the ED and the OR. "I can't imagine a better residency to have a baby in than my PM&R residency. I took call from home, worked only a handful of weekends each year, and even had several rotations with built in mornings or afternoons free" (*How to be a Resident With a Baby and Not Lose Your Mind, 12/16/2010*). Dr. Whoo had to lose her balance completely before she and her husband figured out that work was needed to change:

...we finally had to make some very difficult decisions. The first of which was Mr. Whoo quitting his job to hold down the home front (i.e. find it under Mount Laundry and the River of Dust) and be available for our children and family. The second of which was my decision to break my contract (which cost us a bit financially) and find a more reasonable call schedule in a location closer to our family and friends.

—Dr Whoo, "Balancing Act," December 15, 2010

Being a mom has taught me a lot about balance, but not for the reason you may think. My daughter has a gift for balance that was evident when she was a toddler; we were lucky that she was also innately cautious, so she didn't test climbing and balancing until she could do it successfully. We noticed, though, that she fell less than other kids and that she went up and down the stairs the "grown-up" way from the first time she tried. She took her first dance class when she was three and it was love at first tutu. Despite her natural talent, she had to learn to balance. Passé, arabesque, coupé, attitude front, attitude back. At the barre, then unsupported, then with a partner. She works at balance, at holding herself in space for as long as she can.

The day I took her to buy her first pair of pointe shoes, she put them on and got up on her toes for about ten seconds. *Balance.* She continues to work on it, day after day, year after year. She gets up; she falls out of position. She holds it; she drops it. Sometimes she laughs. Sometimes she grimaces. Sometimes she cries. And then she gets back up and does it again.

She balances—for a moment, for a minute, for a space in time—and then she falls out of it, and she does it again.

Life's successes are defined by expectations. I generally succeed in my professional life, often because my expectations are that I will escape the house without child clinging his banana smeared hands on my newly pressed pants. I'll get to work relatively on time, check my boxes in a timely fashion and make it home in time to let the nanny go. But I almost always fail in my personal life. Maybe because my expectations are those of earlier days when I could balance everything. Maybe because I always forget the take home points of pediatric behavior- you can't make a kid poop, eat or sleep- no matter how hard you try. Maybe my desire to be a "normal" adult is something that is unattainable. I have to learn that while maybe professionally I can do most everything I set my mind to, personally, I can't do it all. And I have to forgive myself for that. And maybe my next vacation means staying at home and doing nothing. I can underachieve once in awhile.

—Jersey, Vacation "Over-Achiever," May 29, 2008

Balance lives in our minds. Balance lives as the ideal serene, unharried, well-groomed woman presiding over angelic children at play and offering up-to-date, evidence-based care to grateful patients. Those images haunt us. They're not real, but they haunt us.

Let's face it: working moms have a lot on their plate. A patient recently complained to me how guilty she felt because she couldn't be a perfect mother, wife, accountant, and friend, all at the same time. If she felt really good and strong in one area, she was slipping in another. "No matter how much I try, I'm a failure!" she declared.

Okay, look, despite the expectations on us, no one can achieve perfection 100% of the time. No one is going to excel in all of the areas of their life always. But we can manage. We can do our myriad jobs well enough. And we can be happy.

—Genmedmom, "How Do You Do It All? (i.e. The Art of Being Imperfectly Perfect)," October 8, 2016

Doctors aren't very good at being imperfect. You don't get through all the schooling and training and competition required without pushing yourself and expecting the best. We were premed. We needed As. We often got them. And now, in the age of Pinterest and butterfly cupcakes and organic clothing, we want to get an A in mothering as well as an A in medicine, and no one is grading on a curve. We don't know the rules before we start.

One of my colleagues sent her kids to the same preschool that my daughter Eve attended. She also had a nanny, so her kids only went to morning preschool; they didn't go back downstairs for lunch with the "day-care kids." (Don't get me started on the segregation). My friend turned to me one day and said "How do you stand it, knowing your daughter has to eat lunch downstairs?" I stared at her. It had never occurred to me that "eating lunch downstairs" = "failure as a mom." My kid was happy, she actually ate her lunch (and often her friend Cassidy's lunch as well), and I picked her up every afternoon. In that community, for a certain group of moms, good moms didn't send their kids to daycare. Preschool was different. Preschool was laudable. Apparently, having a nanny was also OK. A whole afternoon in a (licensed, well-staffed, safe) daycare? Not OK. I was not doing it *well enough*.

My own mother walked into that same daycare for the first time and said, "I thought this would be inhumane, but it's really very nice."

How did doctors before us manage? I was born in 1960 and I'm a third-generation doc. My grandfathers and my father were, of course, men. My dad took call 24/7/365 for the first 8 years he was in practice. He was also the school doctor, the Chief of Cardiology at the local community hospital, and a staff cardiologist at the county hospital. He worked 7 days a week, although on the weekends he was usually home by lunchtime after making hospital rounds. He read newspapers, books, and magazines, had an active social life, volunteered with the local Heart Association, kept up with the medical literature, and attended all our performances (we were theater kids, not soccer players). How on earth did he do it? Admittedly, he didn't need much sleep. But he also, of course, had a wife.

My mother didn't work for pay outside the home until I graduated from high school, and even then it was very part time. Mom wasn't a stay-at-home mother; there were no SAHMs in the 1960s. She was a wife and mother, and "wife" definitely came first. Mom was responsible for making sure Dad's life went smoothly. Mom did all the banking, took care of the cleaning, grocery shopping and cooking, and hired people to do the things she couldn't (Dad didn't mow lawns). Mom dealt with the dry cleaner and the insurance agent and the DMV and the mortgage company and our school. My father read library books every week and never went to the library; Mom did that. Dad wore clothes and never went shopping; Mom did that. Mom also made cookies from scratch, sewed our costumes for school plays, and produced authentic flan for dinner parties. Mom was Pinterest before there was Pinterest.

And so I grew up. I wanted to be a doctor like my dad. I went to med school and started residency, and along the way I married a man who didn't want me to stay home and take care of him. David was perfectly capable of taking care of himself—he could cook and clean and sew and mow the lawn. And yet I found myself feeling anxious and guilty when he cooked or cleaned. Turned out that I expected myself to be a doctor like my dad and a wife like my mother, and that combination simply wasn't possible.

> *In theory, I believe that working mothers are a good role model for children, that fathers step into the home more when a woman works which adds more for the children, that mothers make excellent workers and doctors, that workplaces need to support working parents and indeed workers without children to achieve a happy balance but why can't I shake these feelings of conflict? Why can I think my way to balance but can't feel my way?*
>
> —Jess, *"Guest Post: The Two Kinds of Mothers in Medicine," January 6, 2014*

We still talk about "working mothers" when we never talk about "working fathers." We still think of balance as a woman's issue. Even when we include men in the conversation, it's still a family issue. It's our responsibility to figure it out and make it work despite the external expectations.

> *In my short five months I've been a mom, I already know that yes, I love my job and I love being a doctor but I was born to be a mom...The guilt kills me every single day...family will always come first.*
>
> —Geri, *"Guest Post: A Hard Decision," July 9, 2013*

Many of our writers and commenters assume guilt is the normal condition for mothers in medicine. I never experienced mommy guilt. I was told I would—I was warned that I wouldn't want to go back to work after leave that that it would be oh, so difficult to leave my precious baby in daycare and that I would worry about missing all her "firsts." Maybe my kid was just accommodating; she took her first steps in our kitchen with both of us watching. I know "dog" was her first word, but I honestly don't remember if I was there when she said it or if my husband told me about it. She obligingly said it again, over and over, so that was OK. No guilt. I hadn't missed anything except a few extra dirty diapers and hours of (to me) excruciatingly boring toddler play. Eventually I started to feel guilty that I didn't feel guilty, and that way lies madness.

It's not just "mommy guilt." Many of us also feel "doctor guilt."

...the day I went back to work [after maternity leave] I was 100% ok. I enjoyed it, actually. I felt like I was back at my second home with my second family. The first night back I assisted with a crash c-section and had a blast...I love having every other day off. After a crazy clinic day it is nice to have the next day to decompress. After having a day of playing with my daughter and being at home I look forward to the fast paced environment of being at work the next day...I love both of my jobs. I know my daughter is in good hands...I miss her when I'm working a 24 hour shift but that's not the same thing as feeling guilty that I'm not there. I don't know if it's because I'm the primary breadwinner or some other reason. I am 100% at peace with my decision to work. What I have felt sometimes is doctor guilt. I think part of this is because I was 32 when I gave birth so working is what I've known my whole life. I wonder if I should be working when I'm playing with my girl. I wonder if my colleagues are jealous that they don't get more time off to spend with their kids. (They never say anything - I just wonder). Maybe we'd all be better off as doctors, moms and dads, if we had the flexibility to have more time with our families.

—Anonymous, "Guest post: Doctor Guilt," August 21, 2014

Maybe we'd all be better off.

Flexibility comes up a lot when we write about balance. Many of us work part time, as I did for seven years. Others prize their academic jobs for the ability to time-shift and do some writing or research task "off-hours." We look for flexible child care—the mythical daycare with no late fees, Mary Poppins for our nanny, the delightful au pair who brings enrichment and bilingualism into our homes and does the kid's laundry, too. We also benefit when our children are flexible.

We are, after all, the real constants in the lives of our children. We will never leave them, and we feel confident that they understand that. With my new job and husband's now-reduced travel schedule, we are usually home together with the children by 5:30. Will they remember the changes in their care providers? I doubt it. Will they remember that we were always there for them? I certainly hope so.

—Fat Doctor, "Flexibility is Key: Change is OK," September 16, 2010

My dancer works on flexibility, too. This doesn't come as naturally to her as the balance does. It took her months to work up to a "real" split; it was painful and difficult. There's a lesson there, too.

> *I am constantly pulled in two directions (career versus family) and wonder if my ambition is ever questioned. On the one hand, I don't want to draw attention to the fact that I am very much pulled in these two directions and must balance work and life. But on the other hand, I do want to draw attention to this struggle to help support other women and help others understand decisions working moms need to make.*
>
> *The fact is that I make very conscious decisions that incorporate both my work ambitions and my motherly ambitions...as a working mom, I never want to compromise other women by having my ambition questioned.*
>
> *But even with these doubts, I am incredibly proud of the difficult career decisions that I and every working mother have to make. I know I will only have a short time with my kids at home and I want to cherish that time. I'm sure there will be time in the future to turbo charge my career if I want.*
>
> —Doctor Professor Mom, "Girls Don't Cry," June 23, 2015

One of our guest posters did exactly that.

> *Our profession demanded a doctor be available and on call at all times, so I eagerly offered my services to cover evening, weekend and holiday duties as these were times when my (mostly) male counterparts, who had already put in a long work week, preferred to be home with their families. During the week, my days were filled with diaper changes, making baby food, cooking meals, school drop off and pickups, baking batches of homemade biscotti for the PTA fundraisers and staying on top of the pediatrician appointments, homework, play date and activities schedules. On the days and evenings that I worked my husband took over the child rearing and I headed to the hospital to give expression to that other part of my core identity, that of being a physician.*
>
> —Dr. S. "Guest Post: Tales of a Hybrid Doctor/Stay-at-Home Mum—Part I," March 24, 2014

That all sounds great—until both kids get a stomach virus while her husband is overseas.

> *In the still of the night, they are both asleep. Our house has been vomit free for the last eight hours and the situation appears to be under control. Yet, as I stare at my face in the bathroom mirror, I feel surges of anger gathering up from within me. My children being sick had demanded that I be home with them all day, a duty that I fully accepted and was also loathed to delegate to anyone else. Still, hour after hour of not being able to eat, pee, or shower without being interrupted by a child's need or demand combined with the lack of sleep and extra chores, generated by the sudden vomiting attacks, has all taken its toll.*
>
> *Most of all, I resent my husband's absence from today's circus...travel had become an integral part of a work life that took place in a global village where competition was omnipresent.*
>
> —Dr. S, "Guest Post: Tales of a Hybrid Doctor/Stay-at-Home Mum—Part I," March 24, 2014

Oh, do I get this. I had that moment; it was only one kid, and she wasn't sick, but both dogs came down with acute diarrhea when my husband was away. I had to take a day off work to take the dog to the vet and finish cleaning up. Somewhere in the chaos, my daughter had a bowl of dog food fall on her head (I had put it on top of the refrigerator). Ten years later, she still reminds me of that evening—but we both survived.

Dr. S survived too, and five years later, things had changed:

> Today I work "full time" (whatever that means!) in what is probably my dream job: a perfect mix of innovative clinical care, cutting edge research, medical education and being a leader in my chosen specialty. I am on faculty at one of the most prestigious medical schools in the world and get to work with the brightest and the best, in an environment that is intellectually rewarding and super collegial. ...and I feel this is just the beginning!
>
> My husband and I have never been closer and more happier in our marriage—we are both fulfilled in our careers, but most importantly, feel like we are reaping the rewards of our hybrid parenting model now: family life is fun, filled with endless bliss and joy.
>
> —Dr. S, "Guest Post: Tales of a Hybrid Doctor/Stay-at-Home Mum—Part II," April 14, 2014

One of the crucial pieces of information here is *five years later*. It gets easier for most of us as kids get older. They don't need the same kind of intense supervision; they can feed themselves, wash themselves, do their own laundry, and help around the house. They sleep through the night. Our guest poster advises us to be patient, hold to our values, take the long view, invest in ourselves, remain connected to the reasons we went to med school in the first place—and one more thing:

> Don't pay too much attention to labels, "working mum"; "stay at home mom"; "part time physician". Don't be defined by these terms, they undermine the complexity and power of who you are as an individual. You are unique, you will find a way to make it all work.
>
> —Dr. S, "Guest Post: Tales of a Hybrid Doctor/Stay-at-Home Mum—Part II," April 14, 2014

We struggle with balance, we feel guilty, and we seek flexibility. If we are lucky—and wise—we also find acceptance. The most popular work-life balance post on Mothers in Medicine came from our second work-life balance topic week in 2010. In "Ten Guidelines for Work-Life Balance," Fresh MD (Martina Scholtens) advocates acceptance, boundaries, communication, and reflection.

Accept that you can't have it all—at least not at once—but you can have a life that is rich and full and satisfying... *I'm the mother that arrives late to the preschool Christmas potluck and sets a box of mandarin oranges next to the homemade cheesy noodle casseroles. My son's school uniform pants are embarrassingly short and I couldn't make a recent cross-cultural mental health conference because I'm home with my daughter on Thursdays. But I have kind, secure children and what is arguably the most delightful, rewarding patient population in the city. It's enough.*

She tells us to set boundaries on both our work and nonwork lives. I love her advice for those of us who have a hard time saying "no" in person: "If I feel awkward saying no to someone's face, I say I'll consider their request. Then I say no by email." Perfect. Once we set those boundaries, we can refresh ourselves with writing—one of her prescriptions—and short-term projects that give us a sense of accomplishment.

Several of her suggestions focus on our attitude rather than our tasks. Number three: Don't compare your finances to others. "[N]o good comes from seeing that my family physician neighbour bills more than five times what I do. I start to gauge the wrong things in terms of money; what are quiet days at home puttering in the yard with my four-year-old worth?"

We're all tired. We can reframe our fatigue. This one really made me think:

Consider exhaustion the state of having given, rather than having been taken from. *A few months ago...I thought with dismay how overwhelmingly fatigued I was. I felt drained, spent, exhausted—and reflecting on these words I realized that resenting others having taken from me was passive and inaccurate. I had given what I had by my own choice. When considering Dr. William Osler's words, "Let each day's work absorb your entire energy and satisfy your widest ambition," anything short of collapsing into bed completely spent each night feels a waste.*

The final guideline resonates with me: Marry well. "[My husband] is supportive, a non-complainer, hands-on with the kids and flexible around gender roles. We've both made sacrifices. He is undoubtedly the linchpin to my current contented state of mother-doctor. " There's that flexibility again. We've broken through a series of glass ceilings, and yet we often accept that idea that women must be the primary parents in heterosexual families, because we are naturally more nurturing, or we can multitask more effectively, or because men don't "see dirt." If men don't see dirt, that's because they were allowed to grow up without being held responsible for it. It's not encoded on the Y chromosome. Trust me. I'm a doctor.

David and I have renegotiated the division of responsibilities at least annually since Eve was born. What's his schedule? What's my schedule? What's her schedule? How will she get to dance class/rehearsal/the movies/the mall? We talk about all of it—who will cook? What will we eat? Each of us has some tasks that are only ours. I do the banking and deal with the insurance agent and the accountant and with

Eve's doctor's appointments. He does home and yard maintenance. Everything else—cooking, cleaning, laundry, car maintenance, grocery shopping, helping with homework, calling the school—is divided based on time, energy, and interest.

Our lives will not have balance until men do more of the domestic work. We need to expect it, and we need to allow it. He doesn't pick out matching clothes for the baby? Let it go. He won't do things the way you do, and that's almost certainly OK. If it's not OK—if he's really putting the kids at risk—then work/life balance is the least of your problems.

Fresh MD offers us advice on how to maintain the relationship and the balance:

> *Hold an AGM [annual general meeting] with your spouse. Once a year, {we} hire a baby-sitter and take an evening to take stock of where we're at in every major area of our life: his work, my work, finances, church, where we live, parenting, friendships. We identify what's working, what needs to change and when we need to reevaluate. We like to feel that our choices are deliberate; we don't want to float up to our forties to say, "Huh! So this is how we live."*

Choices. Deliberate. This life is not something that happens to us; we didn't fall down the rabbit hole and end up in Wonderland with a medical degree and a diaper bag. She concludes "I'm a mother in medicine by choice. I accept any challenges and restrictions inherent to this position, for this is exactly where I wish to be."

We are pulled. We stretch. We bend. We work. We get up on our toes, we fall over, and we get up. We laugh, we grimace, we cry, and we do it again. Balance.

Chapter 7
Sharing the Humor in Being a Mother in Medicine

Freida McFadden

My daughter Mel has been going through her "toddler word explosion" lately, so one word we've been trying to teach her is what I do for a living.
Husband: "Mel, what is Mommy's job?"
Mel: "Diaper!"
Me: "Great, she thinks I'm a diaper."
While I am not employed as a diaper, it should be noted that:
Diapers and I both work at night as well as during the day.
Diapers are white; I wear a white coat.
Diapers and I both get crapped on a lot in the course of our duties. (I said DUTIES.)
So my job actually does have a lot in common with that of a diaper, but I am not, in fact, a diaper. Nice try though, honey.

I wake up to a sound in the middle of the night. Beeper or baby? Beeper or baby? Seems like there should be a clear difference. But at two in the morning, for one disorienting moment, it's hard to tell.

Beeper. It's the beeper.

That's better. Possibly better, but potentially worse. Someone could be paging me to ask me about something I could take care of from my bed, whereas baby crying necessitates leaving my warm little womb. Examples of hospital issues I could take care of from my bed:

- "Doctor, your patient can't sleep. Can we give him some Ambien?" (Note irony of waking me up to complain someone else can't sleep.)
- "Doctor, your patient has not had a bowel movement in four days." (… and this could only be noticed and reported at two in the morning.)

F. McFadden, MD (✉)
Mothers in Medicine, 2300 Eye Street Northwest, Washington, DC 20052, USA
e-mail: fizzziatrist@gmail.com

© Springer International Publishing AG 2018
K. Chretien (ed.), *Mothers in Medicine*,
https://doi.org/10.1007/978-3-319-68028-6_7

– "Doctor, we want to report an abnormal urine osmolality." (I swear, I actually got woken up for that once.)

This page, however, is something different. It's an outside hospital calling me. Me—the resident on a *rehabilitation unit*. At *two in the morning*. I'm baffled.

"Dr. McFadden?" a young male voice says on the other line.

"Yes…" I say.

"I'm Dr. Awake. We have a patient here who I think might be a good candidate for rehabilitation," the doctor tells me. "We were wondering how we could transfer him over to your hospital."

"It's two in the morning," I say.

"Well, we were just wondering about the *procedure* for transfer."

"It's two in the morning!" I repeat. There might have been a swear word in there somewhere. I can't honestly say there wasn't.

When Dr. Awake realizes this is going to be a fruitless conversation, he reluctantly gets off the phone. But I have to get out of bed anyway because since having a baby, I generally can't go through the night without a bathroom break. (Baby or bladder? Baby or bladder?) Then when I get back to bed, I'm too angry to sleep. How could that idiot call me in the middle of the night to ask me such a nonurgent question? How inconsiderate!

Well, I console myself, *at least it will make a funny blog entry.*

And that's how I got through residency. No matter how awful my shift was, no matter how many tears I shed, no matter how many times I wanted to throw my beeper out the window (or flush it down the toilet—either way), and no matter how much I missed my young daughter, it always seemed a little better after I came home and wrote about it in a way that would be entertaining to others.

After all, if you can't laugh, you'll cry.

Probably one of my greatest gifts is being able to find humor in life. When I was in grade school, the other kids used to determine the comedic value of a joke based on whether or not I would laugh at it. If even I didn't laugh at the joke, it was definitely a dud.

My "gift" was noticed and appreciated by friends and mentors alike. When I interviewed at one hospital for residency, the interviewer noted, "It says in two of your letters that you have a good sense of humor." He paused. "That's weird."

"Why?" I asked.

He frowned at me. "You don't *look* like you're funny."

"Well," I said, "saying I have a good sense of humor probably just meant that I thought *they* were funny."

Am I right or what?

The time I wrote the most was during my intern year—probably the worst year of my medical training. Aside from the fact that it was my first year as doctor, which is always a hard transition, I was working at a county hospital, where half my patients couldn't speak English and the other half were substance abusers who landed themselves in the hospital thanks to their own (repeated) bad choices. On top of that, I had moved to be closer to my husband, and was now thousands of miles from all of my family and friends. On top of that, my very first senior resident was a woman named Alyssa (not her real name) who seemed to have a personal vendetta against me.

One of my favorite stories about Alyssa took place when we were on call for the Intensive Care Unit. It was actually my second rotation with Alyssa as my senior resident (it seems a little unfair that anyone should get that lucky twice). We had been working for about 6 hours straight when Alyssa looked up at the clock and noted, "It's a quarter past one. You should go get lunch."

I was, of course, starving. During internship, I was always either starving or stuffed so full of junk food that I wanted to hurl. So I raced to the cafeteria before it closed, got a sandwich, scarfed it down, and then returned to the ICU, where I faced Alyssa's blinding, inexplicable rage.

"WHERE WERE YOU?"

I blinked at her. "I… was getting lunch." I added, "You told me I should go get lunch."

"I told you that you could *get* it," Alyssa growled. "I didn't say that you should *eat* it."

Apparently, Alyssa wanted me to buy the food before the cafeteria closed and stash it away somewhere (perhaps in the hollows of my cheeks?) to eat at a later date. Like when I finished internship.

Not to say that Alyssa's antics didn't make me miserable on a daily basis. But it made me feel very slightly less miserable that I knew she'd given me a hilarious story to tell. I drew a cartoon about that incident with Alyssa, and I later wrote an entire novel dedicated to one of the most unpleasant people I've ever had to work with in my entire life. Writing that novel probably saved me several hundred hours of therapy.

At the end of the hardest year of my training, I got pregnant. Soon after, I embarked on the hardest year of parenthood thus far: the first year of my first child's life. I'm sure that when my kids are moody teenagers, I will look back and shake my head dolefully at my naïve younger self, but that was a rough year. For example, did you know that babies don't sleep much? I knew it, but I didn't *really* know it, you know? Not until I brought home a newborn baby that was screaming for milk every hour the whole night.

And when they do sleep through the night per the baby sleep book definition, that really just means they slept 5 hours in a row. So if your baby goes to sleep at 10 p.m. and wakes you up at three in the morning, your baby slept through the night. Hooray, your baby slept through the night! Why do you look so tired?

So I started to plan out a humorous blog entry in my head: which is worse, having a newborn baby in your house, or doing overnight calls every four nights?

Why being with your baby at night is better:

- *You love your baby. You probably don't love your patients. You might not even like them. There's a chance you might hate them.*
- *You don't have to put on pants.*
- *Sleepy husband is probably easier to deal with than cranky residents.*

Why doing q4 at the hospital is better:

- *It doesn't hurt your nipples. (Only your soul.)*
- *Presumably you're doing a job that you love. (Maybe? Possibly?)*
- *They only own you every fourth night. The baby owns you eternally.*

It was soon after that first difficult year that I started blogging for Mothers in Medicine, which was my first time airing my experiences in a public arena. I realized that I had to be careful who and what I wrote about, since I sort of (sometimes) wanted to keep my job. Still, it was hard not to complain. *Everything* seemed unfair back then—I didn't see my baby enough, I worked too hard, I didn't get enough maternity leave, and everyone kept having chest pain when I was trying to pump my breasts. The only thing that kept me from sounding entirely bitter was keeping a sense of humor about my experiences.

For example, while working in clinic one day, a male resident commented to me, "Is there, like, a law that every woman has to have a photo of her baby on the back of her ID badge?"

Instead of getting irritated by his comment, I said, "Well, we can't put it on the front of the badge, can we?"

Then I wrote about how I became one of the many, many physician/mamas who sported a photo of my baby on the back of my ID badge. It covered up the instructions on what to do in case of fire. I don't see women with babies on their badges anymore, so maybe it was just a fad, like legwarmers. But I loved the way my badge would flip around, so that instead of displaying my own photo, name, and job description, I would walk around the hospital with a photo of a baby on my chest. (The epitome of professionalism.)

And then I catalogued the most common comments received by patients upon seeing the photo. It usually wasn't along the lines of: "Your baby girl is beautiful." It was more like:

"Aw, how old is your son?" (Girls are allowed to wear green, you know!)

"Isn't that ID photo of you a little outdated?" (Ha ha.)

"Wow, you have a kid too? You must be exhausted." (Yep.)

As my daughter got old enough to be interested in things that weren't my breasts or a stupid rattle, the first thing I wanted to buy her was a doctor's kit. My husband and I would take her to Toys R Us and gaze wistfully at all the cool toys that we wanted (her) to have. I wrote the following blog entry:

On our latest trip to Toys R Us, I was practically slobbering over a toy doctor's kit. And it wasn't just a doctor's kit... it was a doctor's kit for GIRLS! Now you ask, what made this kit specifically for girls? Why, it was PINK, of course. There was a little pink stethoscope, a little pink BP cuff, a little pink syringe, a little pink otoscope, and a little pink thermometer. Unfortunately, it was for ages 3 and up. (Although the "and up" probably didn't go all the way up to 30 years old.)

Me: "And look! It comes with a little pink doctor's bag!!!"
Husband: "Do you want to buy this for Mel or for you?"
Me: "Ooh, there's a pink penlight too! Do you think it actually shines light?"
Husband: "You know, you have real versions of all this doctor's equipment."
Me: "Yes, but mine isn't pink."
Also, I'm missing my otoscope. Tell me, how hilarious would it be if I were examining a patient's ear and I pulled out that little pink otoscope? Answer: very.

When I finished residency, my daughter was finishing her terrible twos, and there was a brief period when life was easy. But at the same time, the relative paucity of problems in my life didn't inspire me as much as my previous hectic pace. Luckily, that didn't last long—I got pregnant again a year after finishing residency.

They say that having a second child quadruples your work. For me, it only doubled my work. Thank God, because that was still a lot of extra work. And because both kids were in daycare, we were plagued with constant illnesses. To the point where I didn't want to call in sick when I was sick, because if I did that, I might as well have quit my job entirely. I shared the plight of my frequent illnesses with the world:

> *I wake up at 4AM feeling nauseous.*
>
> *I'm not that surprised. My girls have been vomiting all weekend. Not just vomiting—epic vomits. Like the kind where they vomit a lot and you think, "Wow." Then they vomit again. And then a third time. And now it's on the couch, the carpet, the TV, basically everywhere in a 50 foot radius. And then just when you think this may never end, they burst into tears, because vomiting makes kids cry.*
>
> *And they want a hug. But they're freaking covered in vomit. I mean, you have to hug them, of course, but you have to at least attempt to strip off some of those vomit-soaked clothes first.*
>
> *I get this horrible sense of foreboding, but I somehow manage to fall back into a restless sleep and wake up later with my alarm. I still feel really nauseous and my stomach kind of hurts. But I get up and force myself to take a shower.*
>
> *The daycare serves breakfast till 8AM, and I think I'm going to make it. We arrive and as I bring my littlest into the toddler room, I see a bunch of one-year-olds sitting around the table with little bowls of food. But I don't see the food cart. "Can she still get breakfast?" I ask.*
>
> *"Sorry, you're too late," they tell me. It's 8:01AM.*
>
> *"Is it possible for her to get any food at all?" I beg. "She didn't want to eat before we left." And keep in mind, if you tell me "no," I may vomit on you.*
>
> *They seat her at the table and say they're going to try to scrounge up some food. If they're deceiving me, I don't even care anymore.*
>
> *I end up going home sick after my boss takes one look at my face and orders me to go home. But then at home, I try to vomit in the toilet. I can't. How can I be home if I'm not actively vomiting? Now everyone is going to think I'm an unreliable mom.*
>
> *My husband comes into the bathroom while I'm sitting on the floor by the toilet. "Maybe I should have worked today," I say.*
>
> *"I can't tell if you're teasing me or if you're really insane," he says.*

Throughout my career, I always used humor as a way to color my less than pleasant experiences. But I swear that I didn't only use writing as a vessel to share my complaints. Even the best moments in life benefit, in my opinion, from a humorous twist.

Recently, I had the opportunity to teach my younger daughter's preschool class about being a doctor. Sometimes I think that part of the reason I became a doctor was just so I could get to do that. In any case, if you can't find humor in giving a lecture to a bunch of four-year-olds, then you are dead inside.

I was nervous. I'm not sure why I was quite so nervous, considering in retrospect, I can't honestly think of anything that could have gone wrong. It wasn't like I was lecturing to a bunch of Harvard professors—these are individuals who pick their noses and eat it. In public. On the stage during their Christmas show. This was the least discerning audience of all time.

I started out by introducing myself and asking the kids, "Do you know what a doctor is?"

One kid's hand shot up and I called on him. "A doctor gives us s-----," he announced.

I couldn't make out the last word he said, so I took a guess. "A doctor gives you socks?"

The kids burst into hysterical laughter. He said "shots." How did I not know that? That is literally the only thing children know about doctors.

I had this brilliant idea to bring in a pile of rubber gloves for the kids, so they could each put on a glove and feel like a doctor. Except this turned out to be the worst idea of all time. Kids are apparently unable to put on gloves on their own. Several teachers had to be recruited to help. This ate up, like, 10 min.

After that, I had the kids listen to each other's chests with my stethoscope. They came up in pairs of twos so I could help them. Except about a quarter of the class was completely deaf.

Child: "I can't hear anything!"

Me: [adjusts stethoscope] "How about now?"

Child: "No, nothing."

Me: [able to literally feel small child's heart pounding with my hand on the diaphragm of the stethoscope] "Um... sorry?"

Then I broke out my reflex hammer. You want to hear something sad? I actually bought a new reflex hammer just to use in my daughter's class. The fact that I was using it on patients wasn't motivation enough, apparently.

The teachers looked a little nervous about that hammer. Understandably so.

Soon after, we ran out of time, which was a shame because I was just getting into it. The teacher asked the children, "Do you have any questions for the doctor that aren't stories?"

A boy raised his hand: "I went to the doctor and I got a shot."

"Questions that *aren't* stories," the teacher clarified.

A girl raised her hand: "My mom took me to the doctor and I got a shot."

And it just sort of went on like that.

Of course, my older daughter got jealous, so I had to repeat the experience for her class. If I was nervous doing that presentation with preschoolers, I was a hundred times more nervous doing it with third graders. My daughter's teacher actually had to say to me, "Don't be nervous. It will be fine."

And it *was* fine. Afterwards, the kids wrote me cards to thank me. This was my favorite: "Thank you for coming in. If you didn't come in, we would've been doing work. From, Jake." Then Jake drew a bunch of balloons, for some reason.

As I progress in my career and become more concerned with privacy issues, it becomes harder to write about the real humor in being a mother in medicine. I don't feel comfortable telling true stories about patients I've seen recently, even if it's really, really funny that my patient just told me he protects his house with an alligator. (Presumably his home is surrounded by some sort of moat?) And I don't want to spill all the personal details about my children on a public website. Despite my use of a pseudonym, I have no delusions that any motivated person could easily find out who I am.

I still share the humor with my friends and family, and even my older daughter can appreciate some of my funnier medicine-related stories. But in some ways, I don't need it anymore. When I was struggling to get through my early years of training while raising a young child, I needed to write to get through the difficult days. It was therapy for me. I'm grateful I discovered how therapeutic writing could be, and I hope other young physician mothers have the same realization.

Because like I said, if you don't laugh, you'll cry.

Tips for Keeping Your Sense of Humor as a Working Mom

1. You may be spending all your time juggling home/work balance, but avoid the temptation to *actually* juggle your kids. But if you really must do it, start with two kids, and once you master that, you can try juggling three kids. If you can juggle five of them, you may be able to quit your day job.
2. It's fine to let your kids watch television for 1 hour or even 2 hours a day so you can decompress, but letting them watch more than 24 hours a day is not only irresponsible, it's impossible.
3. It takes 11 muscles to frown and 12 muscles to smile, but it takes 40 muscles to laugh. Do it a few times a day, and you can skip the gym!
4. It can be a time-saver on a busy morning to dress your kids the night before. You may also want to feed them breakfast the night before. You probably shouldn't drop them off at school the night before, but if you do, be sure to leave them with a warm, nonallergenic, down blanket.
5. If you buy a crockpot, it can save you a lot of time for meal planning and has only a 63% chance of never once being used and becoming a storage receptacle for your children's small plastic dolls.
6. Avoid the temptation to compare yourself to other mothers who you think are doing a better job than you are at balancing work and motherhood—you are doing just as good a job as any one of them! Well, except for Julie. Julie seems to make everything look so easy and is never stressed out, and did you see the way her girls are always dressed in matching outfits? Man, I wish I could be more like Julie.
7. Be sure to wash your hands thoroughly before and after pumping breast milk. Sterilize all your pumping equipment before and after use. Store your expressed milk in a refrigerator less than twenty minutes after pumping it. Also, swap some of it out with the cream in the break room fridge, because that will be *hilarious*.
8. Whenever you are feeling really down because your kids won't stop screaming or you've been up all night nursing a colicky baby, just remember: only 30 years till retirement!

Chapter 8
Embracing the Mother in Medicine's Village of Support

Miriam Stewart

My daughter has the most beautiful relationship with her daddy. They have their own little songs they sing together, bedtime rituals, games only they understand. She's his little buddy and I love to watch her chat with him in her little 3 year old way about her day or her thoughts. I'm currently on a very long night float rotation and my little one is having a hard time keeping her sleep schedule. Many nights my husband declares that she is going to bed at 8pm on the dot. I often find her snuggled up with my hubby in bed after they've stayed up late watching "one more Dora" or having a jam session in his studio. There is so much beauty in their father daughter relationship. It is deep and substantial and real. I hope their strong bond continues as she gets older and helps her to continue to be strong and self assured. My husband and I love raising this beautiful girl together.

A few weeks ago I was talking to a fellow resident (and mom of 2) about the typical mommy guilt involved with being a resident and spending time away from your kids. She's struggling about choosing a specialty and worried about the damage a more rigorous specialty would cause to her kids. Somehow we got to the topic of her husband having to comb hair and she mentioned that her daughter actually prefers her daddy's more gentle approach to her mom's attempts at taming her hair. And then we starting talking about all the daddy daughter bonds both of our daughters have and reflected that without their busy mamas, our daughters may not have had the opportunity to form these strong attachments.

My daughter is proud of my work at "the doctor house." The time I spend with her is my most treasured and I think our relationship is amazing. How awesome is it that she also has just as enriching and fulfilling a relationship with her daddy. And, I'm not suggesting that dads never form close relationships with their daughters in all other work-life situations. However, just think of how many women you know who report troubled or complicated or loose ties to their fathers. Maybe our girls would have formed all these same attachments no matter what careers we had. But, on those days of horrible mommy guilt, it's nice to think of my baby girl and my hubby dancing, singing and rocking out to their own song.

—Cutter, "Daddy Time," March 7, 2014

M. Stewart, MD (✉)
Perelman School of Medicine at the University of Pennsylvania,
3400 Civic Center Blvd, Philadelphia, PA 19104, USA
e-mail: stewartm2@email.chop.edu

© Springer International Publishing AG 2018
K. Chretien (ed.), *Mothers in Medicine*,
https://doi.org/10.1007/978-3-319-68028-6_8

There is a lot of discussion out there about whether or not women can "have it all," meaning a satisfying professional career and a satisfying home life including partnership and parenting. Five years into my working parenthood journey, I still haven't decided where I stand on the question—some days I feel like the balance between my two primary roles makes me better in each, other days I feel like I can't keep going one more day with the scheduling chaos and the mommy guilt and the sense that I am never quite doing enough in any domain. But what I know to be true is that even if you can "have it all," you cannot do it all. Patients and children have needs around the clock, and it just isn't possible for a person to meet all those needs, all the time, all by themselves. We need help. We need to share the work. This may seem like a self-evident truth, but as women and doctors and parents, we are triply at risk for feeling like we have to do it all ourselves—and do it all perfectly. The cultures of femininity, modern parenthood, and medicine each contribute their part to the myth that you should be able to single-handedly meet everyone's needs—at the expense of sleep, health, and your own sanity if necessary! If you want to be happy in the long term as a doctor-mama, you need to challenge this assumption whenever it arises, either in interactions with others or in your own mind. Let's practice saying it together: "No one can do it alone!" "No one can do it alone!" "No one can do it alone!" Or to use the African proverb made famous by Hillary Clinton in the 1990s: It takes a village to raise a child.

It is easy to internalize the popularized concept that a mother should be "The Only One." The Only One who knows where the lost teddy bear is. The Only One who can kiss the boo-boos and make them better. The Only One who can cook broccoli the way the baby likes it or braid hair or make Teenage Mutant Ninja Turtle pancakes. I don't deny that when these "Only One" moments come up in my household, a secret blush of pride and validation washes over me. It feels good to be the Only One who can sing my daughter to sleep.

Except, I'm not always there, and so for my child it is much better for multiple soothing voices to be able to sing her to sleep. Having a village to help you raise your child not only benefits you—it also benefits your child. As Cutter noted in the above post, the demands of doctoring open up opportunities for our children to have strong relationships with other adults. What is stronger, a table with one leg, two legs, three legs, or more legs? Each trusting relationship your child develops is another source of support and stability. The first step in embracing the mother in medicine's village of support is letting go of the myth of the mother as lone hero.

I spent the first six months of my daughter's life as a quasi-stay-at-home parent. I was in a research year between medical school and residency, and I had the flexibility to be home with my daughter all but two days per week. My partner was finishing graduate school and was often gone from early morning through the late evening. Because I was home much of the day, I hung out with other parents who were not working outside the home, many of whom were practicing attachment parenting, cloth diapering, and making their own baby food. I was ensconced in a world in which two implicit assumptions about parenthood were in play: (1) parents—and especially mothers—are the best answer to almost any question related to their children, and (2) parenthood is the most important role in the life of a parent. It was an all-in culture of parenting, and there was a lot of pleasure in it.

Fast-forward six months. My family moved across the country to a new city, and I started residency at a large and demanding program with a 6-month-old at home. The parenting roles in our household switched overnight. Six days a week I left for work at 5:30 am and often did not return until 7 or 8 pm, so my partner became the all-in parent. I struggled with how to be an all-in doctor, which is what I felt my patients and training deserved, while also maintaining the quality of my relationship with my daughter. The weight of responsibility for the lives of my sick patients was so pressing when I was in the hospital that it was hard to leave, even when I knew that I had an equally important (but less time-sensitive) responsibility to be present in my daughter's life. The standards of parenthood that I had absorbed during my quasi-stay-at-home parent period—which did not allow for competing roles and priorities—left me feeling like a bad mother every day. I cried through my morning and afternoon commutes for months. My baby was in safe and loving hands—spending her days with her other parent, her grandparents, and with trusted caregivers—so my tears were not tears for her, but tears for myself, for the loss of my identity as a "good mother" and the fear that my bond with my daughter would be diluted by my absence.

Since those first painful months of intern year, my definition of parenthood has become much more flexible, and I have redefined for myself what it means to be a good parent. After much trial and error and soul-searching, I have come to the conclusion that as a doctor-mother, I am only as good as the web of connections that I can build and nurture around my family—a web of connections that includes me but can also function without me if needs be for periods of time. This web of connections includes family, friends, paid caretakers, colleagues, neighbors, and members of our community. The village of support has become not only a practical necessity but also a deeply held value for me and one that I want to pass on to my daughter. I do not want her to inherit the dysfunctional mother-as-lone-hero narrative. I want her to know how to build a supportive network for herself; how to ask for, give, and receive help; and how to nurture all of life's important relationships, not only the parental relationship. I am far from perfect in this journey—as I read the words I have written, it all sounds so intentional and well-organized, but in reality it is a well-worn quilt with holes that need patching and many humbling opportunities to acknowledge the ways I could be doing it better. But I am still proud of my motherhood. My daughter and I are deeply connected in a way that no week of service or weekend call can dilute. My job is to stay connected and in tune with who she is and what she needs and to ensure that she is getting the support she needs to thrive—both from me and from the network of other supportive people who inhabit her world.

The village of support extends to the workplace, where the lone-hero model of doctoring is equally problematic. I can't be in the hospital around the clock for days and weeks, so I rely on colleagues at all levels of training to care for patients when I am not there. There are only so many hours in the day, and I can't meet the complex needs of patients by myself, so I rely on nurses, social workers, respiratory therapists, case managers, physical therapists, music therapists, and others to be the village for my patients. I rely on this village to help me honor my commitments to my patients, but also to help me honor my commitments to my family—by switching shifts when my child is ill, getting me out early for a parent-teacher conference, or simply being supportive when there are challenges on the home front.

A Village of Support

As my approach to parenting and doctoring evolved, a post on MiM challenged me and pushed me to even more fully embrace the village of support. AK wrote about sending her child to stay with her in-laws for a month during a difficult rotation for her and her husband:

> A couple of weeks ago, my husband, N, and I found out that we both started our intern year in the MICU. We soon realized that this meant that we would almost never be able to pick our daughter up or drop her off at daycare. Considering it would be her first month ever in daycare, we were stressed! Nanny interviews commenced, and we tried to ignore the impending financial doom that our first month with a paycheck would bring (due to the high cost of nannies).
>
> Soon thereafter, my mother-in-law suggested that we take our daughter, Itty, back home to spend the month with grandparents, aunts, and uncles. Just for reference, we moved 15 hours away from "home, home" a month ago, and we have no family nearby. Initially, I was resistant to the idea, as I couldn't imagine a month without my Itty, but we eventually decided that it was probably the best idea for everyone. Itty would get to see her extended family, who previously provided all childcare for her, and N and I would have a month to focus on our new roles as physicians.
>
> She's been gone for 4 days now. While I was very sad during the first couple of days, I'm now realizing what a great idea it was. Grandparents are happy, Itty is happy (at least for now, she doesn't miss us too much), and we do not have to worry about her at all during a stressful day at the hospital. I had forgotten what it was like to not have to think about picking her up, feeding her dinner, giving her a bath, getting her ready for bed, and putting her in bed. Not to mention the middle of the night awakenings that still seem to happen although she is almost two years old. Once you have a child, it is difficult to remember life without one.
>
> Part of me almost feels badly that I'm enjoying this "me" time so much. I miss her tremendously but also feel that a significant burden has been lifted, at least temporarily. Has anyone ever done anything similar? This is probably the only time that we will ever send Itty away for a whole month, so does anyone have any childcare tips if we are ever in a similar situation again? We were so worried about having multiple new caregivers in such a short period of time, especially with the limited amount of time that she would be able to see us anyway. I can't tell you how many times I've asked myself, "How are we going to do this? What did we get ourselves into? Why did we move so far from our families?" However, I'm confident we'll figure it out, little by little, with a lot of help from others (hint, hint!).
>
> —Anita Knapp, "See you in a month, Itty!" July 1, 2015

I must admit that the post momentarily caught in my throat a little. A whole month apart? It went beyond the place of flexibility that I had managed to carve out for myself around the definition of "good" parenting. But reading the post over again, I let myself really hear AK's voice: *Grandparents are happy, Itty is happy (at least for now, she doesn't miss us too much), and we do not have to worry about her at all during a stressful day at the hospital.* It was a solution that was working for everyone. Her voice was my voice, uncertain but willing to try a new approach, trying to honor all the commitments in her life, hurting but also not afraid to acknowledge the freedom of being able to focus on work without distraction, and most of all, full of love. I have yet to need to be separated from my daughter for a month, but if it were to happen, I would be so grateful to AK for sharing her story. Everyone has to define their village for themselves and find their own comfort level, but I have learned to keep an open mind and an open ear—you never know when you may need to draw on other peoples' wisdom.

In the spirit of shared wisdom, here are some insights I have gained through building my own village of support over the last five years:

Let Go of the Idea That There Is Only One Right Way

I come downstairs after grabbing a few hours sleep in between busy night shifts. I can hear Rose crying in frustration at once again trying to grab the key from the back door. I walk into the chaos in the kitchen. My husband is absorbed in the newspaper surrounded by the toddler carnage. Why is there breakfast still on the table? Why have the pots and pans been pulled out of the cupboards? Has she really got porridge still stuck on her forehead and what on earth is she wearing? Oh and why is she chewing hay from the barn?

I open my mouth to say something but hesitate and hold my tongue. I remember that it's his turn to look after Rose while I am in work mode. We do things differently- I'm the surgeon with the perfectionist streak wanting everything to be tidy and clean; he is the artist and is happy to let Rose run free and wild. I smile to myself.

"Family hug?" I pick up Rose and we all collapse on the sofa together in a warm embrace. A memory to take with me to work that night. Invaluable.

—Lotte, "Guest post: Coming home," April 21, 2014

The people that are helping you raise your child or taking care of patients when you are not on call may not do things exactly the way you might have done them, and that's ok (unless there are true safety concerns, of course). Your partner might have your child sleep in your bed when you are on call, maximizing cuddle time but also raising the terrifying specter of sleep training undone. You may come back in the morning to find that the overnight resident decided to get labs in the morning when you had planned to give the patient a lab holiday. When someone does something differently than you would have done it, train yourself to remember that they had their own reasons for doing what they did, reasons that—like yours—stemmed from a desire to do what was right in their eyes at a particular moment. There might a role for a discussion of your rationale and an attempt to make a plan about the next instance, but you have to choose your battles. No one enjoys being micromanaged or second guessed. Your child will develop their own rituals with each caregiver and will benefit from being exposed to different interests and ways of doing things. Your patients may benefit from a fresh set of eyes thinking about their problem. Let go of the things that aren't truly important.

Be Clear About Your Expectations

The flip side of letting go of one right way is that when there are things that are truly important to you in the care of your children or your patients, be very clear about them with the members of your village. If a sleep routine is important to your child or you want your child to practice the piano at the same time every day, make sure every person who care for her knows the schedule and make clear how important it is. If you want your patient's nasal cannula to be weaned overnight, put that in your one-liner instead of burying it in the sign-out. If you are able to be clear in advance about the things that are important to you and also able to let go of the things that aren't important, you will minimize resentment and conflict while still allowing yourself to feel like you have some control.

Give a Penny, Take a Penny, or Be the Change You Want to See in the World

You know those little change bowls that used to sit next to convenience store cash registers that you could dip into if you were a few cents short? A parallel system exists in the community of working parents. When someone else needs help—a shift trade to attend a child's ballet recital, a last-minute daycare pickup—consider yourself lucky when you can be the one to help! Throw in that penny. You will need to take more than a few pennies back out over the years, and you will feel better about it if you have also contributed. Create a safe space in your workplace for people to talk about the challenges of working parenthood. Give and receive support and help.

Don't Forget to Figure in Your Own Needs

This is one example of advice I can give but still have a lot of trouble acting on myself—it's ok to include your own needs in the list of things you need help to accomplish. I will hire childcare to cover my work shifts, my partner's work trips, family events, and date night, but I find it hard to pay someone to care for my child so that I can write or have coffee with a friend. Suddenly the cost that seems necessary in every other instance seems like an extravagance, and I feel guilty for being away from my child for yet another 2 hours since I already work so much. Over the long term, though, you have to invest in your own well-being or you will burn out, and no one who relies on you will benefit from that. I recommend scheduling a child-free, work-free time for yourself at least once per month. Ok, time to start doing that myself!

Honor Your Partner's Need for Support

The dynamics of shared parenting can make it feel like your partner is your chief competitor for life's most valuable resource: time. If you try to achieve equity by pure numbers of hours of leisure and childcare and paid work and hobbies and sleep and socializing, you will never be satisfied, because the columns will never be truly equal in any given week or month. The attempt to even the score can be even more destructive if there is a disparity in income between the partners, and one partner's time at work is more lucrative than the other's. To avoid falling into this trap, I try to think about what is most important to me and to my partner and how to organize our lives so that we can both have adequate time for the most important things. On a given weekend, I may only need an hour for coffee with a friend, while my partner may need 8 hours to finish a project. You have to make peace with honoring your partner's needs for support as much as your own needs. It is easy to see your work meeting at 6 pm as necessary while viewing your partner's work meeting at 6 pm as a nuisance that could have easily been avoided, but nothing good comes of that kind of thinking. Both people have to trust each other enough to be able to withstand unequal shares of time in the short term in order to feel equally fulfilled in the long term.

Be Smart About Outsourcing

Periodically I become slightly less graceful about the juggling act of my life and end up crying on the phone with a friend about how I just can't do it anymore. Inevitably, the conversation turns to how I might outsource more of my responsibilities. More childcare. More housecleaning. A grocery service. These suggestions are prudent and well-reasoned, and I should probably take every one of them, but there are some of life's tasks that my partner and I want to do ourselves. My partner likes to grocery shop and cook, and so while a service like Blue Apron would save time on paper, it would leave a hole where a core family activity was. We should probably take a grown-ups-only vacation more often, but I have made a commitment to myself that my child will not have to compromise her desire for my company any more than is absolutely necessary as a result of my work. Plus which, our budget is already tight, and there are things we want more than less housework. These are only my examples—yours may be opposite or different. Outsourcing can be a lifesaver, but make sure that you keep your priorities in mind as you decide how much of the work of your home to give away.

Be Generous, Ethical, and Kind to Your Childcare Providers

I am always flabbergasted when people brag about how little they pay their nannies. Before going to medical school, I worked as a nanny for 2 years for a lovely family, and I can tell you that being well-paid and having your personhood acknowledged goes a LONG way when you are managing two irrational screaming toddlers or holding the puke bucket for someone else's child. I want my babysitters to feel that their time and expertise are valued and that they are uniquely seen and appreciated as part of our village. When they are leaving their house to come to mine, I want them to feel good about it. I pay on the high end of the local babysitting rates, offer them free access to our food, and am quick to express my appreciation and gratitude. I am clear with them about my expectations and try to build a long-term relationship. There is absolutely nothing more valuable than a childcare provider who you trust and your child loves. When I leave my child in the care of a long-time babysitter, I harbor no worry or guilt, and I would pay almost any hourly rate for that!

Do Not Judge

Before I had children, I remember having lunch with a friend who told me that she was going to keep her son in daycare during her vacation and use the time to read and reconnect with herself. I thought to myself, "Wow, I would never leave my child in daycare during vacation," but as it turned out, I did that for all twelve of my vacation weeks during residency. It was the only way I got through those years—riding the wave of those quiet afternoons at coffee shops with my laptop and my own mind. If nothing else, parenting has taught me the futility and foolishness of judging other people—as soon as a judgmental thought pops up in my mind about another person's parenting, I bookmark it, because inevitability I will find myself doing that very thing soon enough. The voice that judges others is also the voice of self-judgment. Train yourself to meet the trials of others with a heart of compassion.

Invest in Community

Community looks different for everyone, but no one achieves meaningful participation in a community without investing some thought and time. When you choose where to live, where to send your children to school, where to worship, and where to work, keep an eye out for signs that you could form mutually supportive relationships there and then invest time in forming them. Even though life is crazy and there is no time, volunteer to be on a committee at your child's school or join the neighborhood gardening club or whatever it is that sparks your passion and offers the promise of getting to know people in your community. Take the time to have substantive conversations with neighbors, co-workers, and your child's teachers or caregivers. Building community takes time—I moved to my current city 5 years ago and am just this year feeling like there is a web of connections that could catch us if we were felled by an unexpected setback. When we moved here, I had to fill out a contact person on my child's daycare form in the event that my partner or I could not be reached in an emergency. At the time, I couldn't think of a single person in our city and ended up penciling in my parents who live two hours away. Now there are many families who I would feel comfortable listing, who would pick up my daughter, dry her tears, and take loving care of her in my absence. I am comforted every day by this sense of community and wouldn't trade it for (almost) any salary increase or juicy opportunity in a faraway place!

Express Gratitude

The writer Anne Lamott has said that there are three essential prayers: "Help," "Thanks," and "Wow." In her conception, these are three ways of addressing a divine being, but for me these simple words are equally powerful when addressed to friends and loved ones—the three core gestures of relationship. If you want to build a thriving support network—if, like me, your whole existence has been made possible by the support of others—you cannot spend too much time reflecting on your good fortune and saying thank you, thank you, thank you. As I was reading through the MiM archives in preparation for writing this, I came across one of my own pieces that I hadn't remembered writing, which sums it up pretty well:

It's a good day to be thinking about gratitude. I just got the results of my Pediatrics boards and, mercifully, I passed. Like many things in the life of a working mommy, the whole boards process felt fragmented, stuffed into the crevices of an already packed schedule. I studied in stolen hours, early in the morning, late at night, during E's naps, during quiet moments on call. There existed the dream of reading the textbooks cover-to-cover, mastering the seemingly random landscape of dysmorphisms and eponymous genetic syndromes, committing to memory, not for the first time, the detailed physiology of the nephron. Instead, I did as many practice questions as I could and read all the explanations and made a stack of index cards that I only had time to review once before the test. Studying certainly helped, but what carried me through the process were my patients, the hundreds of people whose stories constitute my fund of knowledge. The symptoms they had, the way their bodies looked and felt under my hands, the labs and images I reviewed in an attempt to understand them, the medicines we prescribed, the way things turned out. All the babies whose birth weight I guessed just before putting them on the scale. All the toddlers who scribbled, babbled, stooped, and recovered during their well-child visits. How do I remember Hurler's syndrome? I remember A, from my first year as a clinical student, and his mother who carried him everywhere in her arms even at the age of seven, because she could not afford a wheelchair. In the boards review study book, they used phrases like "coarse features" and "macroglossia," but I just remember his face, whose beauty became more apparent to me over time, and all the grief and tenderness in his mother's voice as she sang to him, more effective than any medication at calming his agitation. I can only hope that what I have given is somehow proportional to what I have received.

The medical path – and especially the parent-in-medical-training path – has been much harder than I expected and when I reflect on this path I chose, gratitude isn't always right there on the surface. But when I opened the Boards score report, it was right there. I looked up from the computer and the first thing I saw was my spouse. I thought to myself, "How can a person be so steadfast in the support of another?" I am in awe of it. I was the one who first brought up the idea of having a baby in my last year of medical school, before starting residency. I spelled it out to her over the Formica table in our then-kitchen – how we would have an infant while I was taking 24 hour calls and working long days, how it would be an insane juggle. She said, "That seems like it's going to be really hard." But it felt like the right time. We gambled and got a jewel, our daughter E, who is infinite light and delight. But it has been harder than hard. Over the last three years my spouse has done breakfast, drop-off, and pickup almost every day, dinner and bedtime too many days, whole weekends, whole weeks, whole months, sick days, unexpected call-in days, holidays. She gives our daughter what I wish I could be giving her when I'm not there, and so much more. She gracefully bolsters me in my mommy role even though I spend less time with E, when I can imagine a different person laying claim to the "parent-who-knows-more" position. She keeps us well-fed, keeps our household functioning, and through her eyes, I feel beautiful and powerful every day. She does all this while navigating her own full career as an artist and teacher. She has sacrificed some of her own creative and career advancement over the past three years so that I could forge ahead. I know it is painful for her at times – not what she signed up for, even though she did (good love isn't as simple as they say) – but her loyalty and support just keeps shining and it lights my way and keeps our family warm.

So there are many layers to the gratitude I am feeling on this, the first day of the rest of my professional life. Gratitude to my patients, who are my teachers, who have accepted my inexperience and given me the gift of their trust and allowed me to participate in their lives in a profound way. Gratitude to my spouse, for everything. Gratitude to my parents, which is a whole essay in its own right, the years of patient attention and thoughtful decision-making, late night high school research paper crisis management and SOS babysitting saves, self-sacrifice and deep concern for my well-being. Gratitude to my friends, who have stuck with me through long silences. Gratitude to my colleagues and attendings, for saving my ass and helping me find my voice and for caring so much and taking great care of patients and teaching me by example. The African proverb "It takes a village to raise a child" has become so cliché at this point as to have almost lost meaning, but I'm thinking today about the village that raised me, and no words of gratitude are adequate. I will have to thank them by trying every day, with the best of myself, to be of service to the world.

—m, "It Takes a Village," November 22, 2015

Chapter 9
Navigating Life Challenges as a Mother in Medicine

Elizabeth Ann Seng, Dawn Baker, and Kathleen Y. Ogle

> I am the epitome of imperfection. A few years ago, it would have killed me to admit that. Now it is freeing. I am free to embrace my true feelings around life situations. I get mad, I get sad, I get happy. My children experience this, the messiness of me and my life, whereas before I was a shell of a human being covering up all my emotions. I think this allows them the freedom to express themselves as well, warts and all.
>
> I created this, supported by friends and family. The good and the bad. It's not perfect, it's perfectly messy. But there is something amazing underneath. Perfection, bah. Toss it out. Until you do, you cannot fully embrace life; because life is imperfection. When you accept that notion, all you Type A MiM's or future MiM's out there - that is when life truly begins.
>
> —Gizabeth Shyder, "Imperfection Trumps Perfection," April 29, 2013.

We have brought three voices to this chapter to discuss three challenges that women doctors and mothers aren't always comfortable sharing: infertility, divorce, and financial hardship. While some of us have experienced more than one, none of us has experienced all three. We feel that in order to do justice to each topic, a person who has faced that challenge should author the piece. And while I feel like I could write a book about divorce, as I'm sure PracticeBalance and Emeducatormom

E.A. Seng, MD (✉)
Baptist Health Medical Center, 9601 Baptist Health Dr, Little Rock, AR 72205, USA
e-mail: gizabethshyder@gmail.com

D. Baker, MD, MS (✉)
University of Utah School of Medicine, 30 N 1900 E, Salt Lake City, UT 84132, USA
e-mail: mail@dawnlbaker.com

K.Y. Ogle, MD
George Washington University School of Medicine and Health Sciences,
2300 Eye Street Northwest, Washington, DC 20052, USA
e-mail: katogle@gmail.com

© Springer International Publishing AG 2018
K. Chretien (ed.), *Mothers in Medicine*,
https://doi.org/10.1007/978-3-319-68028-6_9

feel about their respective topics, here we offer up a condensed version in order to open up some difficult conversations. I joined Mothers in Medicine before my divorce and blogged heavily throughout on all topics of medicine and motherhood, including a few on divorce. I have to credit this blogging forum and the feedback I received from readers in helping me get through my hard times, and I hope that anyone facing any of these challenges or others not discussed here can find a creative outlet for a release from their emotional roller coaster.

The shame that often accompanies those of us experiencing these issues can cause us to hide our problems from others. We have all found that by sharing our difficulties, not only on the blog but also with friends, family, and colleagues, we have encountered enormous amounts of support that we never would have dreamed was waiting for us. We hope that anyone who finds empathy or solace reading our stories feels empowered to seek support from others and realize that you have absolutely nothing to be ashamed of. Whatever struggle you are going through, you will come out stronger on the other side.

Elizabeth Seng (Gizabeth Shyder)

> *Out of suffering have emerged the strongest souls; the most massive characters are seared with scars.*

—Kahlil Gibran

Infertility

Dawn Baker (PracticeBalance), anesthesiologist

> *I'd learned of it in medical school but never thought I'd have one. I looked for it all throughout my pregnancy, staring down along the midline of my gravid belly. Some telltale signs were there - the nausea, shortness of breath, tender breasts, swollen feet... But I never developed a huge, round, glorious belly that announced the joy of impending birth. Even with the twisting movement of a fetus anxious to emerge, it was hard to believe that this was all real. After years of wanting, of shots and procedures and waiting, it was finally here. But would she come out ok? What would she look like?*
>
> *Then one day she arrived and they placed her on my belly, now saggy from where she was growing. She was beautiful, and I was immediately in love. Nothing else mattered. The nurse came into the room and announced, "It's time to mash on that uterus, shrink it back down!" It was then that I saw it: a faint, fine, dark line running from my belly button to my pelvis.*
>
> *It's the tattoo of motherhood, one I never wish to erase, but I know they usually fade after birth. For this year, it's a gift to me from my daughter. A most perfect Valentine.*
>
> —PracticeBalance, "Linea Nigra," February 14, 2016

Coping with infertility is physically and mentally taxing for any woman, let alone a woman in medicine. Dedicated time, financial resources, and mental fortitude are prerequisites, and all that energy applied to infertility diagnosis and treatment may or may not produce a baby in the end. Women are having children later in life, whether the reason is pursuit of career aspirations, travel, or riding the asymptotic curve to financial security. This truth is never more evident than in our chosen field, where more and more of us are taking the long road of training to become physicians. Unfortunately, advanced maternal age on its own is a root cause of infertility, and it is a significant factor that can reduce pregnancy chances in the face of other infertility problems. This was my situation—a diagnostic odyssey lasting many years, followed by an infertility treatment journey complicated by being old.

It started in the middle of my anesthesiology residency. Even though I was older from having a previous career, I also couldn't imagine giving birth to a child during my training. While we all know women who carry this off successfully, it was just not in my self-vision. But I wanted to be ready for when the right time did come, ideally in 1 to 2 more years. Only I hadn't had a period in several months. My bleeding decreased in frequency during my intern year, but the situation had turned into full-blown amenorrhea while I was working hard and not paying attention. I kept procrastinating the workup, chalking it up to the stress of residency. On the heels of my 35th birthday, I finally saw a reproductive endocrinologist, who recommended some testing. In a complicated and long chain of events lasting over a year, I was eventually diagnosed with a large pituitary adenoma. The tumor was removed surgically, leaving me with very limited pituitary function. The recovery was slow and required me to take some medical leave, and I finished my residency 6 months late.

At that point, I chose to focus my efforts on healing my own body and mastering a new regimen of hormone replacement for not only my reproductive organs but also my thyroid and adrenal glands, all the while knowing that my chances of ever becoming a mother now were pretty low. I pushed those longings aside, studied for and passed my board exams, and secured myself in an attending position. Then one day my husband told me he wanted to try for a baby. I burst into tears, overwhelmed with the thought of having to use reproductive technology to get pregnant. As I suspected and later came to realize, it is not for those with faint of heart or lack of resources. The average IVF cycle in the USA including the necessary procedures and medications costs approximately $15,000, and it is rarely covered by insurance. Not only does each pregnancy attempt take a significant portion of a year (during which a woman's eggs are undergoing the natural process of aging and DNA damage), but each cycle also requires quite a few appointments for monitoring, lab draws, procedures, etc. Due to the unpredictable nature of egg maturation during the IVF stimulation, cycles can be canceled at any moment. Not to mention the risks of multiple gestations, ectopic pregnancies, and ovarian hyperstimulation syndrome.

We decided to try it, knowing that it was truly our only chance at giving birth to our own child. My life became consumed with cycles of daily injections and transvaginal ultrasounds and 2-week waiting periods. And yet as one of the newer partners in my group, my internal allegiance would bounce between hopes of success and duty to my work schedule and patients. I had to take a lot of vacation time, and I did quite a bit of begging for shift swaps when each cycle culminated in an egg retrieval or embryo transfer procedure. Doctor's appointments and operating room schedules don't exactly mesh!

The first egg harvest was a screaming success: lots of eggs retrieved, and on my first embryo transfer, I got pregnant! But before the joy could even sink in, that little heartbeat on the ultrasound was gone. I had not been shy about sharing my infertility journey with my coworkers because they all knew about my pituitary surgery. I wished I could take back the numerous pregnancy disclosures I had made, but it was too late, and the awkward conversations accumulated. We moved on after a D&C with frozen transfers from the bank of eggs I had made. Months passed, I underwent three frozen transfers. The scheduling, the shots, the procedures, and the life on hold… no pregnancy, and then the bank was empty.

My husband had tried to console me with (flawed) logic. "Think of it as one long pregnancy," he said. "I mean, all the eggs were retrieved and fertilized on the same day. It's like they're all part of the same process." He could never quite understand the despair of the early miscarriage, the sadness over that glimmer of what could have been, now made worse by the subsequent failures. All things IVF had become my hobby, my pastime. I put my athletic pursuits on hold due to exercise restrictions during the cycles, and I said no to travel opportunities. And *the babies*! Friends and coworkers had their own babies left and right, passing me by with their family achievements. I felt unlike myself, and I felt unwomanly. It was difficult to accept that I needed so much assistance achieving something that is so basic to human life as reproduction. After our bank of embryos was gone, the watershed decision was before us: do we keep going? How many times do we do this? How many times *can* I do this?

With the help of journaling, meditation, therapy, and lots of talks with my husband, I chose to continue with another egg harvest, this time incorporating preimplantation genetic embryo testing. Being a healthy athletic woman, I had underestimated and ignored the statistical reality that at 40 years of age, my eggs contained a significant amount of DNA damage that only worsened my fertility odds. This additional testing was offered to me from the beginning, but I was initially in such a hurry to get pregnant that I didn't want to spend the extra amount of time or money that each cycle required for the freezing and sequencing. I wish I had listened more closely to the statistics the first time.

Around 4 years after the diagnosis and removal of my pituitary tumor, I became pregnant. At first I kept it very secret, and I was always worried that something would go wrong. But I stayed pregnant, and in the end, I gave birth to a beautiful baby girl at age 41 in the hospital where I trained, where I was treated for the cancer that caused my infertility, and where I now continue to work.

For a while I thought I wanted to help other women by writing extensively about infertility—the realities, my experiences, my lessons learned. Yet after years of consuming my life, it has now become something I don't think about. IVF wasn't the most horrible experience in the world, but subconsciously my mind wants to avoid those memories. The image of my daughter's face blunts any pain that might surface, along with the fact that I'm now a busy physician mother to a high-energy toddler. One lingering thought is that becoming a patient when you are also a doctor changes you as a person and a physician. It makes you better at both endeavors. Illness is a great equalizer; you realize when climbing into the stirrups of the procedure table, or being wheeled on a gurney through swinging doors into a drafty operating room, or lying in a lumpy hospital bed with nothing on but a crisp, cold gown that you are no better than any of the other patients fighting for their health and dignity around you. As an anesthesiologist, I now love providing my services for procedures in the IVF clinic. As a person who went through the IVF process, I am grateful for the self-care tools that I was forced to explore and identify. Infertility will challenge your personal relationships: friendships, family bonds, and romantic relationships. There can be differences in opinion on direction of care, number of IVF attempts, or ethical issues with genetic testing/embryo selection/possibility of multiple gestation/etc. Everyone has different preferences for ways to deal with stress, but here is what worked for me:

- *Journaling or blogging about my experiences.* I have always loved to write and find it to be an easy way to sort through my feelings. Discussing some of those feelings on a blog also proved therapeutic and helped me to connect with people who had experienced similar feelings—either related to infertility or other challenges.
- *Doing some sort of formal meditation.* I cycled between yoga practice, walking, gardening, acupuncture, and guided meditations during my IVF journey. When I did my injections, I made a relaxing ritual out of it using music, cold packs and heated massage as necessary, warm tea, and the occasional dark chocolate peppermint patty. Again, preferences for these modes of stress relief can be very individual, but luckily there are many resources to choose from.
- *Accepting the situation.* There were lots of times when I didn't feel like myself because I wasn't following my normal routines related to exercise or work. I wished I could "go back to normal," being a goal-oriented high-achieving professional, but then I realized that my normal had shifted to a new, primary goal of getting pregnant. Other endeavors—rock climbing, lifting more weight in the gym, taking on a new certification at work—took a secondary spot in my list of priorities.
- *Talking.* In addition to connecting with others through my blog, long talks with those close to me—in particular, my husband—became very important for processing thoughts and plans of action. He left the final direction of our infertility journey up to me, but we worked through all the decisions together extensively. At one point, however, it became important for me to also talk to an objective third party. A counselor helped to provide a sounding board when I was trying to figure out my boundaries for how far I would theoretically take my fertility treatments.

Would I want to do it all again? No, but I would if it was the only way to get my beautiful baby girl. And I would encourage the use of IVF to another woman in need of its amazing and yet daunting technology. Was it worth everything I experienced to become a Mother in Medicine? Most certainly.

Divorce

Elizabeth Seng (Gizabeth Shyder), pathologist

What will they think of me? The question coursed through my mind like an interrogation. You see, I had crafted a perfect image. Double doctor marriage, two beautiful kids. What was hiding was the fact that my marriage was crumbling—the beautiful exterior hid a train wreck. We had been traveling separate paths for years, me following societal norms of doing it all, chief resident, nursing mother, and caring for toddler. Denying the fact that I was no longer in love with the person I married. By the time I entered counseling, it was too late; a cliché, I know.

One partner's response, a female who has since retired, was like a salve. "Gizabeth, it's going to be ok. 50% of marriages or more end in divorce. My sister is divorced. Half of our partners are divorced. We won't hold this against you, we will support you."

That was 6 years ago. We are in a new place, a blended family, one that gets along 95% of the time, with 5% arguments. I think that's better than most intact families. I got remarried this year, and with hard work and lots of therapy, I think I have crafted a new chapter: something better and with promise of permanence through mutual love, kindness, and support.

If I step back 6 years in time, though, it was very hard.

Divorce sucks. It's not for everyone. I, certainly in my Disney princess fairy tale happy ending view of life and marriage, never dreamed it would happen to me. I didn't know many people who were divorced, although that list has grown over time. My parents are happily married for over 40 years, and that is how I thought all of this was supposed to happen, especially having two kids who were at that time aged 7 and 5. I remember sitting down with my Mom at Starbucks coming from a walled up, stressed out, angry confused place declaring, "I want out." She recommended that I go to couples counseling and start individual therapy. "If not for this relationship, for your next one. You'll keep repeating the same mistakes over and over." It was good advice. Although reinforcing that I needed to get divorced, it softened the blow. I can't say the process was entirely peaceful, but when we weren't emotional, we agreed to stay on the same page, not let the kids split us, and try to make the transition as seamless as possible for the children.

There was a huge learning curve. Hiring lawyers. Answering interrogatories. Doing house inventories. Learning the custody and child support lingo. Taking transparenting classes to learn what to watch for with the kids—how to support them emotionally and make sure they weren't taking on too much of a caregiver role in a single parent home. I remember being devastated to learn I had to give them up for half the summer—we separated in February 2010 and divorced in September 2010. I had terrible insomnia that first summer—constantly worrying over how they were doing without me.

My son, the younger one, was only 5, still an age of magical thinking. He didn't talk about it much, and at first I made the mistake of thinking that it was easier for him. I talked to a friend who has a mother with a master's degree in child development, and she said that girls usually come through it better because they talk more, and boys shut down. I started paying more attention and had to troubleshoot some fear, separation anxiety, and stuffing emotions. But his teacher at school reassured me at the time. "Jack used to sort of exist in a bubble. He was in class, but he did not participate. Since you have separated, he is coming out of that bubble. He interacts more with the other kids, and in class." I almost choked back tears of mixed emotion. Glad that I was doing the right thing for my son and simultaneously realizing that he was mirroring me, in the marriage. For the longest time, I lived in that bubble.

My daughter, the older one (7), was at that age group that likes to play "Parent Trap." She was constantly trying to get us back together, which was heartbreaking to watch. Even though my ex and I were so separate in the marriage, I could see that at age 3 and 4 she was trying to get us together; it was more intense. For example, "Mom, I'm going to have Dad bake you a cake for Mother's Day so you get back together." She got him to do it—she has amazing powers. "Mom, when is Christmas? I want from Santa for you and Daddy to get back together. Can we start writing to Santa now?" How do you respond to that? "Yes, write, that's what I do to get my emotions out," while your heart is breaking because you know that you cannot give her what she wants for Christmas this year.

Fast-forward to the kitchen table at breakfast 2 years later. My daughter says, "Mom, Dad sure does some things really well. He picks good women. He picked you, and he picked Stepmom. She's a lot better for him. She likes steak, and she's ok with him hunting all the time." I laughed. It wasn't easy; it was my son's turn that year to ask Santa to get us back together. I was still stumbling through the monthly bad Match.com dates I forced myself to go on. But we were stable, and I worked hard to support and appreciate my kids' stepmother for taking care of my kids.

One thing I took pleasure in at the time and continue to enjoy is all the freedom that came after years of being a doctor and primary caregiver. Not that there wasn't the excruciating double standard of missing the hell out of my kids and worrying that my absence would mar their future (so far that has not borne out to be the case, I see that they are enriched by having a bonus dad and mom), but oh! Yoga, wine, exercise whenever I want, blog more, brunching and shopping with friends, walking around the house in my underwear until noon, taking long showers, and not worrying if your kid was going to wander off into the street or make a mess or hurt the cat. Of course freedom comes naturally with having older kids who never want to hang around with you on the weekend anymore, but when they are young, it's a pipe dream.

Everyone who goes through a divorce has some personal not-for-public-airing reasons for making that difficult decision. At this point for me, those things are water under the bridge. But I can reflect on some broader societal issues that certainly played a factor in mine. I remember first learning on Mothers in Medicine that other countries don't have such a tough time with work-life balance. Commenters from Australia were horrified by our short maternity leave—mine was 8 weeks. And while magical, those 8 weeks were also very lonely and felt unsupported. Much less a "paid vacation," as one of my male coresidents quipped to me, than a daily struggle of: How do I figure out this breast pump and is this lump a breast abscess that is going to send me to surgery and keep me from breastfeeding my child (thankfully not, reassured my OB) and how do I do this mothering thing and go back to work?

I became insanely jealous of doc/moms I knew who had stay-at-home dads. I grew up in the South and completely accepted the traditional role that I was the primary caregiver. Relinquishing any of that role to my then husband would not have worked in that marriage. But that's a job! And then I had this other doctor job. Both of which I did well but it stretched me to my breaking point, and I slowly built up anger and resentment that poisoned my marriage. I voraciously read articles that beleaguer this issue—it's not unique to doctors. And I think it's changing—as much grief as we give Millennials, they are demanding longer paid paternal and maternal leave, and progressive companies like Facebook are responding. Traditional professions like physicians and lawyers and architects have yet to respond, but the current trends are promising. I think paternal leave should be a norm. If your partner in life is supporting you in this difficult and lonely transition, it can only work for everyone—both bonding with the child and each other.

Even though I'm a few years out and life is stable, the wounds of divorce can be reopened. I follow Mothers in Medicine on a daily basis, commenting on almost every post. We recently got a new contributor who is going through a divorce. I read this blog and ended up having to lock the door of my office in order to keep the pathology lab from seeing my tears.

> *Today, in my boss's office, I reflected on my failure to be this person I aspired to be, and who I thought I was. I also talked about my failure to be the role model I wanted to be for my residents. I humbly asked his advice about how to handle it. It wasn't so much that I wanted his advice on how to handle my divorce and all of the emotional muck that goes with that (it is so deep) but how to negotiate this space where most of my trainees know me as married, two kids, physician, teacher, academic. At this moment, my new identity is single mom with two kids, physician, teacher, academic. And I'm struggling on every single one of these fronts. And frankly, it's hard for me to struggle. I'm a perfectionist by nature – good survival trait for a physician, but it turns out to be a harmful trait when everything in your life goes up in smoke. Poof.*
>
> *I'm noticing that I'm deeply clinging to my sense of self as physician and leader, but I feel this person (or who I thought she was) slipping away. In the last nine months, I haven't lived to my own standard, nor been the person my residents think that I am. So, am I a fake? A fraud? An impostor? Poof.*
>
> *At one point during my talk with this boss, with tears and eyeliner cascading down my cheeks, and both nostrils completely clogged with snot, I said, "I'm fighting my way back. I'm doing the best I can right now (sob, sob), and I know it's not my best. But I'm really trying. And it's super important to me that you know that, and you don't lose faith in me." He sat there. He nodded. And he sat there some more. And I cried a little more. And, you know, like a good primary care doctor, he just let the silence be the space between us for a while. And then he said softly, "I think, really, if I was going to give you any advice, it would be to let go of the concept of fighting to come 'back.' You'll never, ever be back Frieda. You will be somewhere, but let go of the idea that you will be back where you were before. Nothing is ever going to be the same. Poof.*
>
> *And, so it was burned in me, under my skin. These words. This wisdom. It was so right. How come I hadn't thought of it before? In some ways, a liberating thought. In most ways, it deepens my grief. I'm a fighter. A bootstrapper. A resilient woman. I've been putting all my energy into paving my way "back." Literally every ounce of my soul, strength and breath have been put toward getting one foot in front of the other everyday to get back to where I was – and I suddenly realize I've been deluding myself. It's so simple, in fact, but I've just been unable to see it. It begs the question, so just where am I going? Forward? Then what?*
>
> —Frieda B., "Fighting Back," June 10, 2016

Frieda's words were amazing, retelling my tale with a new unique voice adding fresh wisdom to past history. I've been there. You can bury it, but it will still jump out at you when you least expect it exposing the raw wound and allowing you another big cry to aid in your healing. My response in a comment, after I recovered myself: "It's such a hard journey. The 'you' that you are becoming is going to look back on the 'you' now and before divorce and give ginormous hugs because she will be her strongest self emerged. You are heading toward your butterfly, and she is going to be stunning." I hope my kids and my blended family and my friends and relatives look at me and catch a glimpse of that butterfly. Divorce is truly a transformation. Academic intelligence does not equal emotional maturity and self-actualization, but if we work hard, we can achieve it all.

Fast-forward to the present and future. I met a man on Match.com about 4 years ago, and we married this fall. My husband and I shared bread and thanks at Thanksgiving with my ex and his spouse last year. She is a former caterer, which has brought me up to a level beyond the fish sticks and mac and cheese my kids and I subsisted on 6 years ago. I don't hope to compare to her cooking, but my husband and I are learning to cook healthy meals. My husband is very plugged into the kids, with homework and projects and carpooling and emotional support. I see that my kids' stepmom, a fifth grade teacher, is holding my ex to standards I was unable to in the raising of their 3-year-old daughter. Remarriage is exciting. Living with a blended family is rewarding. There is life past divorce. I hope that anyone going through it will read this account and know that whatever future they are headed to can be better than the present.

My daughter, at 13, is excelling in academics and thriving in cross-country, track, and dance. My 11-year-old son is also doing great at school and working hard and achieving in martial arts. They love their mom, dad, stepmom, and stepdad and don't feel the need to compete for anyone's love or to worry about their love being not enough for us. Love and kindness is enough, in itself. It's the foundation for happy relationship and the struts that bring you through the hard times. I know not every divorce can lead to such calm blended family waters, but to anyone unfortunate enough to be going through it, there is a light at the end of the tunnel, and your words, actions, attitude, and sometimes therapy can help lead you to it.

The Cost of Being a Doctor and a Mother

Kathleen Ogle (Emeducatormom), emergency physician

Children are expensive. So is medical school. Children take up a lot of time. So does medical school. Unfortunately time and money are two things in considerable shortage during medical training.

—Mrs MD PhD, *"Money and mothers in medical training,"* October 10, 2016

Isn't That the Truth?

I'd always known I wanted to be a doctor, a doctor and a mother. My journey into medicine, however, was a circuitous one. Part of that has to do with the fact that by the time I came of age to truly consider it, the only thing I knew was that medical school was really long and really expensive. Money was a nebulous and intimidating thing as a result of my upbringing in a setting of limited financial means. I think it was partially due to what many call a "broken home" but what seems to be more of the norm these days. My parents split when I was 2, citing irreconcilable differences and spawning a war between the two of them that held me for years as a pawn.

My father rarely, if ever, paid child support to my mother, who had custody. Dad was career Navy, often deployed for 6 or more months at a time. My mother and I moved frequently, initially bouncing from grandparents to aunts and uncles before I started school. My stepdad, my mother's crush from high school, entered my life when I was 4, and we all moved a fair distance from my grandparents. Money was tight, but somehow my mom found a way to feed us on a limited income. I remember helping prepare meals from a very early age, and any time I complained of hunger, I was told to eat a slice of bread or drink a glass of water. Yum. So satisfying. Our nomadic trend continued, about every 6 months to a year to find the next cheapest apartment, so I rarely went to the same school for long. My studies, however, were of paramount importance to my stepfather from the start of my education. So important that I would be "grounded" if I didn't perform to his dictatorial standards. I often thought to myself, "Well, I don't have any friends anyway, so what's grounding me going to do?" My "teacher's pet" status did nothing for my social success from elementary school through high school. This also meant that I wasn't able to foster long-standing friendships throughout childhood. Home was rough in other ways that do not align with the content of this chapter, so suffice it to say, I was happy to seek positive reinforcement by being a high performer in school. I was also a latchkey kid at 7. I'd walk home from school, let myself in, put on afternoon cartoons, do the chores laid out for me, and start on dinner prep according to the list left by my mother. I would summer with my father on either the Atlantic or Pacific Ocean, during which time it seemed he was trying to compensate for lost time (and not paying child support) by spending money on fun activities or school clothes, most of which came from the women's petite section of select department stores. This led to school clothes being blend of hand-me-downs from neighbors, garage sales, thrift stores, outfits lovingly hand stitched by my grandmothers and my high-end department store fare. Such an awkward blend for my wardrobe palette, and not so good for my social status.

I'm the first in my family to go to college. This means I had very little mentorship in preparation for it. As we lived paycheck to paycheck, I certainly knew I couldn't expect financial help from my mother and stepfather. I knew vaguely of the concept of scholarships, but I didn't know how to advocate for myself in the process and highlight my extracurricular activities in such a way to improve my chances for scholarship awards. I was a good student, but I wasn't an honors student. I wasn't in

AP classes. I knew nothing about how to navigate paying for food, books, living expenses, living in dorms, or any of the other terrifyingly unknown things that come along with undergraduate studies. I knew nothing about grants. I had limited guidance from the high school counselors and was unable to work through these discussions with my parents because they were too busy working. I was hopeful that the lifelong promises from my father to at least pay for my tuition would come to fruition. Those promises dissolved halfway through my senior year of high school when my father informed me that because he'd bought a house and two new cars and was focused on his new family, he wasn't going to be able to help with school. I felt like I'd been punched in the gut. I was angry, hurt, disappointed. I was also determined to make something work.

My study plan at that point in time was to become a psychiatrist. In my mind, a psychiatrist was someone who counseled people, helped them through their issues, and would be easier to achieve than being a doctor. I literally didn't know that psychiatrists were doctors. Ultimately, my mom and I talked it over with my grandparents, and it made the most sense for me to live with them in their small town and go to community college and then maybe eventually transfer to state school when I could get more scholarships. I'm so thankful for them. They let me borrow one of their cars to get to and from classes. They fed me well. They loved and supported me. I didn't have to worry about living expenses. I could focus on school and how to pay for it. I learned about the grants that I was eligible for because of my parents' limited income. I was offered a college credit card application. I was able to pay for my books and my lab fees. I was making forward progress. I found part-time work at Wal-Mart (quite possibly the worst job ever), which ultimately allowed me to save enough money to buy my aunt's old car. 1988 cherry red Ford Festiva, 4 speed standard transmission, my pregnant roller-skate, for $500. I'm sure she gave me a huge deal for the car, but handing over that cash was huge. I'd never seen that much money in my life. Letting it go was really hard, but it was also amazing to have my own car. I had a job that allowed me to pay for my gas, my car insurance, my books, and a little bit of entertainment. I fantasized about being in my late twenties, a flourishing psychiatrist driving my hunter green convertible Mazda Miata down the Pacific Coast highway, wind blowing in my hair.

Now, let's talk more about that focus on psychiatry. My grandparents knew a doctor in our church who had a colleague who was a neuropsychologist. To them, that was the same as a psychiatrist, so they connected me. This woman was brilliant, sophisticated, focused, and successful. I helped her review some charts on the psychological performance of patients who'd experienced traumatic brain injuries of varying severity. Ultimately, she sat me down and schooled me. She let me know the difference between what she did in practice and what she had to do to get there. She also walked me through what it took to be a psychiatrist. It then hit me again, like a ton of bricks. Medical school is really long and expensive, and I have to find a way to pay for it. I ruminated on that for a while.

I wandered the halls of my community college. I noticed postings for the nursing school. My community college had a 2-year associate degree program for RNs.

Hmmm, I thought to myself. If I can get a nursing degree in 2 years, I can get a hands-on glimpse of medicine. I can decide if it's really what I want to do before I dive in. I can also make more money and find a way to save for it. I talked to my aunt who was an LPN. I applied. I got in. Two years later, I was prepping for my board exams. Now, in the midst of all of this, I'd fallen madly in love (in retrospect, more likely lust) with a guy that ultimately wasn't so good for me. He was domineering, dismissive, verbally abusive, but the best sex I'd had to that point in my life. By the time I was graduating from nursing school, he'd joined the Air Force, become stationed in Las Vegas, Nevada, where we'd eloped, and I was pregnant. We were also miserable, and he had orders to move to England for 2 years. He was on active duty and had a regular paycheck, yet I was going to nursing school and working part time, sending him the majority of my paycheck because he needed it. I asked very few questions, but ultimately realized he'd become a compulsive gambler and philanderer. I realized that I could not leave the country with him. He left the country, angry. He and his mother threatened to scoop my child from my arms as soon as it was born. We were still married and I theoretically had health coverage as a military dependent. Because of a problem with the application process, I had to go to the judge advocate general to resolve it, get some financial support from him, and get prenatal care setup, all while I was trying to find work as a new grad RN. That week, I'd also gotten notices from all of the bill collectors in Vegas regarding the bills he'd left behind. I was being sent to collection, because I had no income, no way to pay, and he was out of the country. As I was signing in with the prenatal care desk, I felt a gush between my legs, then running down my legs. I excused myself, went to the bathroom to differentiate between urine and amniotic fluid. This was not urine. I knew my baby was not viable. I knew what this meant. This meant bedrest for the duration of my pregnancy in the midst of being in collections, having no job, having no money. This meant significant potential complications for my baby, even if I made it to a viable gestation. I asked them to induce, to terminate. It took a week, because ultimately, they would not allow me to decide without informing him in England that I was doing so. He took emergency leave and came to "support" me. My first son would be almost 20 now.

Once we moved past the loss of our son, I reflected on our relationship, realized it was most assuredly toxic and terminal. I needed to pull the plug. I ultimately found a nursing job which allowed me to save enough money to move away. I chose Las Vegas because it was halfway between my parents and because I had some friends there from my husband's time being stationed there. I lived with my mom while I worked as a nurse in a home hospice agency. I saved what I thought was a comfortable amount of money, which was about $3500. I packed up my Ford Festiva and hit the road. I found a temporary agency nursing job and got my first apartment. I bounced from unit to unit. I had an air mattress and an alarm clock radio.

I finally got a regular staff position in a medical-surgical step down unit. I bought some dishes at Target. With my first paycheck, I got a TV with a DVD and video player. I felt really fancy. Next paycheck, I got a little table and two chairs. I had the air mattress for about 6 months before I had enough money to buy a bed. I spent about a year and a half on the step down unit. We took care of postoperative coronary artery bypass graft and aortic aneurysm repair patients. We had bowel resections, carotid endarterectomies, femoral-popliteal bypass grafts, and aortobifemoral bypasses. Occasionally we had spillover of stroke patients or other general medical issues. My patients were 1 or 2 days postoperative and had high acuity, mediastinal and pleural chest tubes, Jackson-Pratt bulb drains in their vascular sites, and external pacer wires with external pacemakers. We ran drips on the floor: diltiazem, dopamine, dobutamine, procainamide. We did synchronized cardioversions and chemical cardioversions on the floor. We had post-op patients code, stroke, and bleed. It was intense. It was intellectually stimulating. Because of my drive, I quickly moved up to charge nurse and code team leader. I wanted more.

I moved into the surgical ICU. This meant I was the frontline nursing provider for the previously mentioned surgical patients. I recovered what we called hearts (post-op CABG) directly from the OR. I stripped chest tubes, used autotransfusers, vigilantly monitored blood pressures to keep them tightly regulated, titrated drips, monitored Swan-Ganz numbers, input/output numbers, balloon pumps, and coded patients. I was a night shift nurse. Our hospital was not a teaching hospital, which meant that at night, codes were run by the nurses until the ER doc could make it over to supervise. We were very autonomous. We also had flight nurses in house who could at least intubate, if needed. I was an advocate in end-of-life discussions, I consented people for surgery (informed consent is the RN's responsibility, right? *Sarcasm, of course*), and I intently questioned all of the docs about why they were doing what they were doing. Why are we using levophed instead of dopamine? Why milrinone instead of dobutamine? Why fresh frozen plasma instead of cryoprecipitate? Why femoral access instead of subclavian? I studied their movements when they did procedures, particularly central line and Swan-Ganz insertion. Six months into my tenure in the surgical ICU, I was assisting an anesthesiologist with a Swan. I prepped the patient, laid out all the equipment, handed him the equipment in sequence, anticipated every move. I realized at that moment, I wanted to be the one doing it. The next morning, I sat down with my nurse manager. I told him I wanted to go to medical school. I needed a bachelor's and pre-med courses. I needed to be free during the week. I proposed I work every weekend for the foreseeable future in order to be available for weekday classes. I went to the university to discuss my options. Most of my nursing classes didn't cross over for a bachelor's in biology. I registered for classes. For 4 years, I worked every Friday, Saturday, and Sunday overnight and went to school Monday thru Friday. My university based scholarships on need, not on academics, so though I carried a 3.7–4.0 GPA, I made too much money to qualify. I gulped and took out my first student loans. In the midst of this, I also paid a lawyer $5000 to secure my divorce while my now first ex-husband was abroad. I applied for medical school. I got into three. I was 27. I had wrestled with staying in the same geography with the hopes of maybe making another bad relationship work and maybe have a chance at being a mom. I chose me. I moved to the east coast to start medical school.

For the first time in my education, I decided to just do school. I refused to work and go to school anymore. This was my passion and my dream. This was an investment. I was going to get the most out of my investment, so I look at my medical school loans like a mortgage. This mortgage is going to support me and my family for the rest of my life. Right now, my loans cost more than my rent.

While in medical school, I entangled myself again with a man that wasn't so good for me. Emotionally immature, philandering, noncommunicative, insecure, defensive. It was always a roller coaster of a relationship. I remember being between second and third year of medical school, planning to move in together and he broke up with me. I had a week to find a place. Thank you Craigslist. Again between third and fourth year, planned to move in together, we were on the rocks again and he was fooling around, and I ended up moving in with another friend. We tightened up things during fourth year; he proposed a week before match, knowing full well my match list was not predicated on our relationship. I ultimately matched at my home institution. Spent my intern year planning our wedding. Went through the typical ups and downs of residency. I paid the utilities and groceries, he took care of the car insurance and mortgage. Before my third year, he told me he wanted a divorce. I crumpled on the floor. Pored over Craigslist to find something I could afford. Found a furnished studio. Spent the next 6 months in a deep depression. Didn't talk to him at all. Struggled on my resident salary, but was making it. Started to come out of it and then he came out of the woodworks. "We should get to know each other again. We should date. We should go to couples therapy." We started seeing each other again, and he creeped back into my heart. I found out in March that I'd been chosen to be one of the chiefs. A week later, still living in my studio, still dating my husband, I was running around, emotionally labile, breasts tender, looked at the calendar. I was late. Went to CVS immediately, grabbed a pregnancy test, went to Starbucks to use the bathroom, and found two pink lines. I broke down. I'm a resident, living in a studio apartment away from my husband with whom I have a tenuous relationship, and now I'm about to start my chief year, pregnant. Where am I going to put a crib? How am I going to afford childcare? Called one of my mentors and my OB, made an appointment, shook and cried in her office because I didn't know what to do. Of all of the things I'd wanted in my life, it was to be a mom and a doctor. He never wanted children. Maybe I could do it by myself. It's impossible. Ok, I'll tell him this is his golden ticket. He can walk and I'll figure it out. In the same week, I found out he was still in bed with one of the many women he'd canoodled with over the years. I most assuredly did not trust that he could be a good husband. He'd already proven that. We fought. We discussed termination. I almost did it. I finally talked to my best friend in the whole world, and she basically slapped me in the face over the phone. She said, "What are you thinking? You've never wanted anything but this. You are thirty-four, you are a doctor, you are amazing and you can do this." I cried so much, knowing that she was right.

> *I knew it wasn't going to work. I. Knew. It. Was. Not. Going. To. Work. I felt compelled to give it one last go for the sake of our little one. I also had an inner dialogue that was determined to figure out how to at least be a parent with this man. We made a small person. I'm stuck with him no matter what happens between us and our relationship. I have to tell my child when they've grown bigger and understand more of the world that I did try to make things work. I also had to give my ex the opportunity to be a father, though he never thought he wanted to do that. I wanted to be able to look into the eyes of my pride and joy when they ask why mommy and daddy aren't together and speak frankly, honestly, that I did everything in my power to make things work… and they just didn't. I want to say that we both love our child and have our child's best interests in mind and want them to grow up happy and healthy.*
>
> —*Emeducatormom, "The End…and The Beginning," November 8, 2015*

I often have to remind myself why I chose to go so deeply into debt. Sometimes I wonder why my choices have led me to go so deeply into emotional debt. As I reflect on it today, my little one's father and I are almost divorced. I want to find a mutual ground in which we can continue to coexist and maintain financial and emotional stability for our son. We share expenses, but I shoulder a heavier load. I spend thousands of dollars a year on the convenience of having a nanny to accommodate my clinical and academic schedule and act as the go between him and I on days in which our schedules do not align. I spend money on takeout when I'm too exhausted to cook, and I just want to cuddle my little dude on the couch. Sometimes I spend money on massages and pedicures, and I have twinges of guilt about being so frivolous, given my roots. I've spent thousands of dollars on lawyer's fees. I want to buy a house. At this point, however expensive, however emotionally draining, I'm in a much better place and I'm thankful for my struggles. They've forced me to reflect on practical and romantic aspects of life. When I look into my little one's eyes, hear his exuberant laugh, see his one-sided dimple, hear his father's sarcasm, and bear witness to his zest for everything, I realize, I'm one lucky doctor mom.

Summary

Three unique tales of infertility, divorce, and financial hardship reflect wisdom gained from our struggles, and we know there are many of you out there going through challenges of your own. We hope that readers who can empathize gain knowledge, but more importantly fellowship. The natural tendency is to draw inward, but sharing when you can with whomever you can is so much healthier for your soul. May you find peace and happiness no matter what you face in life.

Chapter 10
Negotiating for the Job You Want

Jane H. Chretien and Audrey P. Corson

The second interview I went on was a large private practice group in the city where my husband practices. It's a group of approximately 80–90 radiologists. We talked about my dual boarding in radiology and nuclear medicine. We discussed the possibility of working within my preferred subspecialties (breast imaging and nuclear medicine). We discussed the possibility of working part time, which got me really excited. I also met some of the radiologists in the group, who all seemed very nice. However, when I came back after my interview most of my conversations with my attendings at work went like this.

"How was your interview?" "Good. I really liked the practice"
"What is your base salary?" "I don't know…"
"What is your retirement?" "I don't know…"
"What benefits are offered to you?" "I don't know…"
"What about maternity leave?" "I don't know…"
"Do you get paid overtime for call?" "I don't know…"
"How many years until partnership?" "I don't know…"

Basically, I felt like an idiot. And now, I am waiting to hear back from both jobs but I feel like I cannot really compare and contrast since I don't know the answers to these questions!

How do you go about asking these questions during a job interview? Do you ask right away? Do you wait until there's a proposal? Is there anything else I should be asking? Do you need a lawyer to review your contract?

—X-Ray vision, "Help with attending interviews!" October 26, 2016

J.H. Chretien, MD, FACH (✉)
Department of Internal Medicine, The George Washington University School of Medicine,
8120 Woodmont Ave, Suite 320, Bethesda, MD 20814, USA
e-mail: chretien.jane@gmail.com

A.P. Corson, MD, FACH
Department of Internal Medicine, The George Washington University School of Medicine,
8120 Woodmont Ave, Suite 320, Bethesda, MD 20814, USA

Florida Atlantic University, Boca Raton, FL 33431, USA
e-mail: acorsonmd@gmail.com

© Springer International Publishing AG 2018
K. Chretien (ed.), *Mothers in Medicine*,
https://doi.org/10.1007/978-3-319-68028-6_10

Everything is negotiable. Well, not *everything*. However, through our long careers in outpatient primary care internal medicine, we have had to navigate many obstacles and realize that negotiation helps overcome these obstacles. As mothers in medicine who have now graduated to grandmothers in medicine, we offer experiences from our career partnership, which we hope may guide you to increased job satisfaction.

Any mother in medicine is smart, hardworking, and dedicated. But these attributes relate to the intellectual attainment and drive to succeed in medicine and to do our best for our patients. The business world is foreign to most of us. Whether it's desirable or not, medicine has become a business. And in business, negotiating is an important skill.

Before making assumptions about your ability to negotiate, just consider that you have negotiated many things in life. You simply did not have the label for your actions. Remember your own teenage years—curfew hours, use of the family car, attending a concert. Didn't conversations with your parents jockey back and forth, with you asking for more than was reasonable and parents caving on at least a few of the issues? Maybe "yes" to the concert, but only if accompanied by several friends; maybe "no," your newly licensed 16-year-old friend will not be driving. So you, the teenager, win on attending the concert and have bragging rights to your friends at school on Monday. You will forget to mention your loss: that transportation was provided by a parent. Your parents won on their biggest issue, which is your safety. They will be driving you home. Their loss is that they regard these large concerts as a waste of time and money and they still worry about drugs. Thus, both sides have won on an important issue and lost on some trivia.

Similarly, anyone with a young child becomes quite skilled at negotiating, if for no other reason than to prevent meltdowns. Negotiating is a life skill that we all possess and most of us are quite adept.

Somehow we don't adapt these skills to our professional life. For those of us entering medical careers decades ago, there was a sense of struggle from the onset, gratitude to have made it, and no inclination to ever ask for anything. Thus, we never considered negotiating. This may change with current female representation in medical schools averaging 50%, but we suspect that women may still lag in asking for what they need and deserve, especially when feeling vulnerable because of pregnancy and raising young children. In fact, a recent study of 10,241 academic physicians at 24 public medical schools found significantly lower salaries for women, even after adjusting for specialty, faculty rank, funded research, publications, years' experience, and Medicare payments (a marker for amount of clinical work) [1].

Since storytelling is a good launching point for retention of a concept, let's start with one of our early stories [2]. We were both employed by the same university clinic when we had young children at home. We had been thrilled by the offer of 50% employment. Everyone knows that in medicine, half-time means 50% pay for at least 75% time. We worked 5 days a week, 6 hours a day in clinic. Outside of those hours, we were responsible for any of the clinic patients who were hospitalized and for after-hours call every other week, 24/7. But the job still looked like a good position in terms of being family friendly. Our children often came along to the clinic on "snow days" or other school holidays. They could watch TV in the hospital doctors' lounge when either of us rounded on weekends. Life was sweet.

But then one of us had a chance meeting with a young male physician from our division at a shopping mall on a Wednesday afternoon.

"Hi, are you on vacation this week?"

"No, this is my weekly discretionary time" he replied.

"Discretionary time????"

"Yes, the day I don't see patients. The time I write my book, review residency training curriculum, do phone conferences…"

Let's calculate this data. He's our age, similar amount of training, hired by the same university division. We, the two female physicians, each work 5 days for 6 hours, or 30 hours of clinic time per week for 50% pay. He works 4 days for 8 hours, or 32 hours in clinic for 100% pay. Our complaints went nowhere. We thought there was nothing to negotiate when we had signed a contract. But in retrospect, we had not analyzed the situation.

And this gets us to the most important point. Do NOT sign a contract without review by an attorney. Not your cousin, the newly graduated attorney returning a favor, not your neighbor the real estate attorney. We mean A CONTRACT ATTORNEY. And not just any contract attorney, but one who specializes in physicians' contracts.

Eventually, knowing we had to leave, we looked at positions in a different division of the medical center. By this time, contracts were becoming more complex, and a 20+ page document was presented for signature. We were still naïve about such matters. We concentrated on what we wanted, which was such trivial items as "8 clinic sessions per week instead of 10," and an extra 3 days of CME time, etc. The contract also included a noncompete clause of 25 miles for 2 years, meaning neither of us could seek active clinical employment for 2 years at any facility within 25 miles of our main hospital OR within 25 miles of any satellite facilities. This seemed onerous to say the least, so we asked legal affairs about making an exception in the contract for government employment. We were told, "No exceptions." Finally, one of us asked advice from a well-respected contract attorney. This turned into an expensive official consultation that was worth every penny. Bottom line: "You cannot sign this contract. You would probably win in a court case, but after exhausting all your savings." Good advice. However, the final punch line on this story, since we already had decided we couldn't sign, is that we, as naïve physicians, initially had all the wrong reasons for not signing. We completely missed the big picture. We missed the forest for the trees, in the words of our attorney. While we were concentrating on clinic hours, we missed entire scenarios in which our work situation could be made intolerable, and we couldn't escape without huge financial penalties.

Eventually we moved together into a different hospital system, and we decided ahead what we needed in terms of work situation. And since our job offer was to work together to set up a unique new satellite clinic for the hospital, flexibility in work conditions would be important. We negotiated verbally for salary and reasonable benefits and threw in some probably non-reasonable benefits as wishful thinking, but who knows what might be granted. Then, when the document was provided to us, we passed it to our contract attorney. He identified the plusses and minuses, and we had him do the actual negotiation on the contract itself. The outcome was great while it lasted. The organizational structure did fold after a few years, but from poor business management by our employer concerning its payer sources. And, our attorney was there for our final bailout.

Certain employment issues cannot be negotiated. Salary offers from government institutions or residency programs, for instance, are usually fixed for all candidates. But if the job is something that you want, look for the additional benefits that would sweeten the deal. On-site childcare? Additional CME time? Assignment of a scribe? (Seems essential to function in the ER). Pregnancy leave? Short-term disability? Some of these items can be negotiated without changing the official salary structure.

Another nonfinancial matter of extreme importance for job satisfaction is the relationship between you and supervisors and between you and lower level employees. First, to whom do you report? Is it the department chairman, the chief resident, or a senior faculty member? You need that information in writing. Many of us have been in a position where the supposed supervisor is the Department Chairman or the Medical Director of the hospital, but really his administrative assistant (a nonphysician) informs you of complaints, supposed transgressions, or changes to your clinic schedule. This seems much more common when administrators are dealing with women physicians rather than with their male counterparts. If X number of patients are required to be seen per day, make sure that this is a standard for everyone at your level. We once had an administrator inform us, "I don't like your schedule template." Never mind that we were seeing larger numbers of patients than many in the group. It was all a power play, which we knew and she knew. As your professional success often depends on your supervisor, it's important to understand what agenda your supervisor has. Based on our many years of experience in practice, we strongly believe that reporting to anyone but a physician will result in dissatisfaction. It's also nice to have in writing that professional issues will be covered by the chairman or some other designated physician.

Also of importance is the issue of you supervising mid-level providers such as nurse practitioners and physician assistants. Remember, you have the medical license; when lawsuits hit, the physician is usually held responsible. Many employed positions now look for one physician to supervise several mid-level personnel, which we feel is difficult, maybe even impossible, to do. You cannot do your own patient care and see every patient of the NP or PA. And for complex illness, you may be signing off on big mistakes. If your dream job requires that you supervise a mid-level, then you need increased compensation or decreased number of patients yourself.

Basic Issues in Negotiations

But let's get back to some concrete basics. You found what looks like your dream job. Before the initial job interview, you need to identify some objective data:

1. What we most frequently identify is the salary. It's useful if you have either a written job listing or insider information from friends as to the numbers. Compare with similar opportunities at other practices or hospitals. Compare with national and regional ranges. Remember our opening paragraphs and the differential payments to male and female academic faculty of medical schools. Know your numbers. If the salary is fixed income, you want a situation of salary transparency. In government positions, this seems to be the norm. But in academic institutions, hospitals, and private practice, there may be a wide range for a given position. You should decide ahead what is your lowest acceptable salary, what is the likely salary, and what is your reach goal. You are in a better position if the first offer comes from the employer, unless you already know the range. In private practice and in some university positions, you are responsible for your overhead expenses. Find out how it is calculated. If overhead is too high, you will almost be working for free. Overhead varies by specialty and by how tightly expenses are controlled. We can speak best to outpatient primary care, where it should be about 50%.

2. Before negotiating, make sure the rewards of the contact are worth the risk of losing the job offer. An experienced business negotiator, George Siedel, refers to always knowing your BATNA [3], that is, your *best alternative to a negotiated agreement*. When you have a strong alternative, you are not desperate. You can converse more easily about what you will bring to the practice and how you expect to be rewarded.

3. Be realistic. For instance, if you know the position offers 5 CME days, you can request 7 or 8 with a good reason, such as attending a special conference that will allow you to institute a new research project. If you request 20 CME days, you lose credibility.

4. What are your expected hours in clinic or in the hospital? Some specialties such as ER may have rigid sign-in/sign-out times. You may get a concrete definition of what is required for full time. Others, typically outpatient primary care, may only define in terms of number of "sessions" per week. As more and more patients are assigned to your "session," you end up with a nonviable work day. This can be described as the hamster wheel clinic, with four to five patients per hour, no matter how sick they may be.

5. What is the flexibility of the work day? This varies all over the map. We interviewed at one prominent private clinic in another area of the country, as they wanted us to set up a satellite in our own area. The concept was exciting, the salary more than acceptable. Then, we found that even a single day's absence required at least three months' advance notice. For those with young school-age children, we can assure you that very few kindergarten performances schedule three months ahead. Do you want to be forced to call in sick for the first grade music concert? On the other hand, in our current small private practice, a physician can take leave as long as there is adequate coverage and if the requesting physician is cooperative about helping out colleagues for their own urgent family matters.

6. See if you can get some idea on turnover in the position. A new physician every year or two is a bad sign.

7. Get to know your "opponent." What is your goal, what is their goal, what might you have as common goals. Negotiation is more successful when you know something about the institution or the practice, when you know the people in charge. While employed by one large hospital, we were asked to justify our salaries, and we were not getting a straight story from the administrators. So, we invited the hospital CFO for coffee and presented our numbers. (Gets back to know your numbers.) We had gathered data on number of patients seen and the payments expected from their insurance coverage. We were also able to define, with numbers, administrative waste in our clinic and give alternative solutions. All in a very friendly, noncombative session. Sometime later, when embroiled in a termination dispute with the hospital, our relationship with the CFO paved the way for smoother negotiations. Getting to know the other side in a personal way is somewhat like business associations that develop on the golf course. In fact, we sometimes regret not having taken up golf!

8. Next, we get to the famous "noncompete" clause. Most employed positions now have such a clause in the contract. Obviously, a hospital or partnership that hires you doesn't want you to spend 2 or 3 years building up a loyal panel of patients on their turf, then see you launch off on your own and siphon these patients away. So, there is nothing wrong with a noncompete that is reasonable. Reasonable time is considered about 2 years. That is, 2 years after you leave, you can open an office or take a job wherever you want, the theory being that by that time none of the patients will follow you. Distance tends to be trickier and does vary with rural vs. urban locations. But a few miles is considered reasonable. When a noncompete clause in an urban environment forbids you to practice medicine for the next 2 years within 25 miles, it has nothing to do with your taking away patients and everything to do with punitive action.

9. Besides the noncompete restrictions, another huge impediment in an exit strategy is your malpractice. Most malpractice policies have what is called a "tail." This is a sum, usually a very large sum, payable when you leave, to cover possible malpractice which occurred during your employment but which hasn't made it yet to a lawsuit. The statute of limitations for lawsuit may not yet have run out when you leave, and thus you may not know anything about the case. Then a year or two into your new job, you get named in the suit. Who protects you? Hospital employment is generally straightforward. The hospital policy covers the tail. But in private employment, unless it is specified in the contract, you could get stuck with the equivalent of a second mortgage! A common fair way of dealing with this is that you pay when you leave voluntarily, but the practice pays if they fire you without good cause. This one item by itself justifies use of a physician contract attorney.

10. Finally, if you don't ask for it, you don't get it. One example that continues to amaze us occurred during an offer from a different hospital. The location was inconvenient for both of us and we demurred. The offer kept improving. Finally, when we said that night admissions were problematic because of dis-

Table 10.1 Common negotiating factors

	Government	Hospital[a]	Private group
Salary/bonus	Fixed	Negotiable	Negotiable
Vacation	Fixed	Negotiable	Negotiable
Sick leave	Fixed	Negotiable	Negotiable
CME time & expenses	Maybe	Negotiable	Negotiable
Retirement account[b]	Fixed	Fixed	Maybe
Insure: health, malpractice	Fixed	Fixed	Maybe
Supervising mid-levels?	Negotiable	Negotiable	Negotiable
To whom do you report?	Maybe	Negotiable	Negotiable
Protected research time	Negotiable	Negotiable	N/A
Hours or clinic sessions	Negotiable	Negotiable	Negotiable

[a]Hospital refers to post-residency employment
[b]Retirement accounts such as 401K usually have fixed guidelines by law

tance and a somewhat unsafe neighborhood, the headhunter actually offered round trip from home with chauffeured car service for any night work! Ask for more than you expect. This is especially true of CME time, CME expenses, professional time, sick leave, and vacation time (Table 10.1). It all depends on how much they want you, and right now women are in a strong position for many specialties.

Mental Preparation and Assembling Your Team

We've been discussing the objective information you need for an employment interview and the factors you need to think about before any negotiation. But also, you need the right attitude for an interview. After gathering the above data on the basics of considering a job or joining a practice, next you need to work on your own mindset before the first meeting. You need to know what you want. You need to know you are worth everything you ask for. You need to be determined and non-apologetic. You need to dress for the interview to project power. You need to be prepared emotionally to walk away from an offer that is bad. An exit strategy is essential. If the noncompete is favorable enough, and the malpractice will not be a detriment, lots of other questionable things in a contract can be accepted, because you know you can escape. And always remember, "It's not personal, it's just business."

Once you think a position will be a good fit for you, you need to assemble "your team." Number one on the list is an attorney, and as we mention several times, an attorney who specializes in physician employment contracts. If you are employed by a large organization, you should also have an insurance advisor. The organization will cover malpractice, but you need to examine your coverage on life insurance, short-term disability, long-term disability, and coverage for legal dealings with the medical board of your state. (Surprise—if a patient makes a complaint against you to the medical board, or a hospital tries to fire you for "disruptive" attitude or whatever they may complain about, your malpractice may not cover legal advice or representation. You may need special insurance. However, in our state as of 2017, this will be included in malpractice.) If you are joining a private practice or want to start your own practice, then in addition you need an accountant and a business advisor. Payment in private practice may not be straight salary. There are all sorts of mechanisms which determine your income based on collections, or complexity of the cases your see, or hourly rates, minus whatever the practice calculates as your expenses, i.e., the amount it costs the practice to support you. These calculations may or may not be fair to you, and basically you need an intricate knowledge of medical billing and collections to see if your income reflects what you earned, thus the need for a skilled business advisor.

After you have accepted a position that is anything other than straight salary, you need to know your numbers. Get acquainted with the CFO of your group. Straight salary is straightforward. But once bonuses are added for performance, whether it's number of patients seen, or income generated, or satisfaction scores, you need to know the rules. In fact, concerning bonuses, you should be satisfied with the salary structure first, because bonuses are often an empty promise.

In summary, when new graduates leave residency for their first attending position, most are clueless about negotiations. This appears to continue into a pattern of simply accepting what is offered when changing positions. Women are more likely to be afraid of serious, businesslike negotiations and try to avoid conflict. Women want to please; they want to have a work situation that is good for their families. It is not necessary to be confrontational. But know your worth. Be positive. Expect respect. Know what you want. The satisfaction of attaining fair compensation and good work conditions allows you to be a better mother in medicine.

References

1. Jena B, Olenski AR, Blumenthal DM. Sex differences in physician salary in US public medical schools. JAMA Intern Med. 2016;176:1294.
2. Chretien JH, Corson AP. Equal opportunity discrimination. Md Med. 2013;14:24–5.
3. Siedel G. Negotiating for success. Essential strategies and skills. Ann Arbor: Van Rye; 2014.

Chapter 11
Question and Answer: The Collective Wisdom of Mothers in Medicine

Rebecca E. MacDonell-Yilmaz

From its first post in 2008, the Mothers in Medicine (MiM) blog has provided a space for sharing anecdotes from the front lines of motherhood and the practice of medicine. It has served as a way for women to support one another and provide guidance, share experiences, and offer a variety of perspectives on navigating the challenges of this cross-section of callings. It has also served as an avenue for women who are interested in pursuing, or who are already in the throes of pursuing, medicine and motherhood. Though each woman's experiences and opinions are unique, certain themes have emerged over the years. The advice offered by the writers of Mothers in Medicine in response to the most common questions and concerns is collected below and reflects the input of women practicing in a variety of specialties and settings, speaking from every point along the spectrum of training.

Can I Have a Family and a Career in Medicine?

This is, with its various iterations and nuances, the most common question posed to the women of MiM and echoes as an undertone throughout the column, its questions, and responses: can I do it? And while each person, preference, and circumstance is unique, the resounding answer, despite complications and caveats, is a resounding yes.

Yes, you can.

While there is no single recipe or golden rule, common themes rise clearly to the surface of the feedback and advice shared through this forum. Below, pearls of wisdom from across the years are synthesized around the big-picture issues tackled most frequently by MiM and its readership. While some of the language refers

R.E. MacDonell-Yilmaz, MD, MPH (✉)
Division of Pediatric Hematology/Oncology, Hasbro Children's Hospital,
593 Eddy St., Providence, RI 02903, USA
e-mail: rmacdonellyilmaz@gmail.com

© Springer International Publishing AG 2018
K. Chretien (ed.), *Mothers in Medicine*,
https://doi.org/10.1007/978-3-319-68028-6_11

specifically to pregnancy and childbirth, most suggestions pertain to raising children in general and apply to parenting in any form, whether biological, surrogate, foster, adoptive, or any other arrangement that leads to loving and caring for a child.

When Is the Best Time to Have Kids During a Medical Career?

Many women begin to ponder this question long before they are ready to dive into parenthood, even before they have identified the person (or donor or support system) with whom they hope to undertake this endeavor. And given the length of training required of physicians in the United States (four years of college, four years of medical school, three to seven years of residency depending on specialty, potentially followed by an additional one to three years of fellowship for sub-specialization), even women who begin medical school as early as possible will find themselves deep into their years of potential childbearing by the time they emerge and begin to practice as attending physicians. And while there are many factors that influence the timing of motherhood that are out of your control, there are notable pros and cons to starting a family at each stage of training. Below is a discussion of the major factors to consider and how they evolve throughout a medical career.

Flexibility of Schedule

Flexibility is a strong point on the list of pros for having a child during medical school. Unlike the subsequent steps in this journey, medical school includes time off during holidays, mostly free weekends, and vacations scattered throughout each year. It also generally affords the greatest amount of flexibility in scheduling; rotations can often be rearranged, and many electives allow for lighter hours that can be especially helpful either late in pregnancy or when returning from maternity leave. Some students extend their undergraduate medical education by taking an entire year away from the standard training to do research or to pursue additional training, including a master's degree or, with a longer gap in training, a PhD. Many schools design their curricula to allow for several months of flexibility during the fourth year for residency interviews, which can also be used for leave if interviews are clustered near the beginning or end of that time period. While some women advise against going on interviews while pregnant due to the potential for discrimination and assumptions on the parts of programs that an applicant might be distracted by family obligations, others have found that being pregnant on the interview trail brings a taboo topic to the forefront and serves as a litmus test for how accepting and accommodating programs might be for parents of young children. In addition, having a baby early leaves more time in the future to space out the births of any additional children (if desired) and, though impossible to eliminate, can decrease the chance of facing age-related challenges with fertility or, at the very least, bring them to light earlier to allow more time for trying to conceive.

Unlike any other phase of medical training, medical school is also a time when absences do not require coverage by another person. The nature of residency and many fellowship schedules is such that house staff are integral to the functioning of the hospital, and in order to maintain coverage throughout the hospital, any resident or fellow must arrange in advance for someone else to cover every shift or call that they will miss during their leave. This can place a large burden on the other members of the training program. It can also present challenges in scheduling the remainder of time in the training program, as most programs have a culture of paying back or making up any shift that is missed or traded to another trainee. Both the size and culture of the program can affect how easy or difficult it is to rearrange schedules and to coordinate coverage.

On the other hand, the reality is that many women do have babies during residency and fellowship. Some take longer maternity leaves and extend their training past their planned graduation date. Others stack vacation time with electives or lighter service months and trade away as many shifts and calls as possible to accommodate a leave. While some women who waited until later write that they couldn't imagine juggling a child with the full-time endeavor of residency or fellowship training, others found that the added challenge led them to be more focused and efficient. Multiple women who had one or more babies during residency note that they still went on to become chief resident.

Still other women prefer to wait until they have completed all of their training before starting a family. Many feel that they would prefer to wait until the time when they have the greatest amount of control over their schedules in order to be able to plan their maternity leave, although the amount of control and coverage will vary widely by specialty and practice setting.

One caveat to any consideration of scheduling is that pregnancy can be unpredictable and complications or a premature or (even slightly-earlier-than-anticipated) delivery can throw off even the most carefully cultivated plans. In addition, there is general agreement that it is best to try to avoid delivering during intern year, which is extremely difficult and exhausting even without a child, and to try to avoid taking any of the United States Medical Licensing Examination (USMLE) steps or board certification exams late in pregnancy or in the first months after delivery.

Partner/Family Support

Even with excellent, reliable childcare, medical training will keep you away from home for long hours, putting additional demands on the other parent or members of your childcare team. The stresses and sacrifices of medical school and training can put a strain on any partnership, just as having children can. The combination of the two is especially taxing, and while it is certainly doable, setting up as much support as possible is always advisable. This can come into play when deciding when to start a family, as your level of control over your geographic location is lower during training as compared to when you enter the job market. Are there several schools or residency programs in the vicinity of relatives who are willing and able to assist with childcare? If so, how competitive an applicant will you be at these programs? Are you or your partner active duty in the military, with the potential of being stationed somewhere far from any of your support systems? These questions can also be important to consider when determining what pathway is best for you (more on that later). Given the extensive number of hours that you will spend studying or working, it is imperative to set up reliable childcare (as well as backups!), to multitask (e.g., studying/eating/making phone calls while pumping if you choose to and are able to breastfeed), and to ask for help.

> Here's a toast to getting by with FaceTime, nannies, dads, moms, friends, support groups, childcare centers, vodka martinis, grandparents, Munchery/Pizza Hut/Whole Foods/ Amazon Fresh – we're getting it done – mothering AND medicine.
>
> —*ZebraARNP, June 8, 2016*

Finances

Let's get right to it: childcare is expensive. Whether you opt for daycare, a nanny, or an au pair, or some combination of these, the costs add up quickly, especially given the long hours for which you will likely need to arrange care. Even if you have a spouse or partner who is willing to be a stay-at-home parent, that still represents a lost income on their part. Living near family members who are willing to help can ease this burden, but it still deserves significant consideration, especially if you are looking to start a family during medical school, when you are not earning a salary. Unless the baby is born near the end of the fourth year, when there is typically a gap of at least several weeks between the end of medical school and the start of residency (when you will once again be earning an income), it will be necessary to arrange childcare for after you return to school. If there is no support system readily available, such as grandparents or family members who will care for your baby for free, it may be necessary to rely on a partner's salary or to increase the amount borrowed in student loans to cover these additional costs.

Greater financial security tops the list of reasons some women advise waiting until after training to begin a family, citing the relief of feeling somewhat settled in a home and a career, as well as the ability to save while making a higher salary in preparation for maternity leave and future childcare.

Ultimately, despite the different challenges that exist at every step of training, most respondents encourage women considering motherhood to do what is best for them and their families regardless of where they are in training. Many note that things often work out the way they were supposed to.

> It's not an easy road, but a rewarding one.
>
> —*Gizabeth Shyder, December 27, 2016*

There's no perfect time, and it will be hard no matter what. But good too, of course. Good luck!!

—Anonymous commenter

I Already Have Kids. Is It Too Late to Pursue a Career in Medicine?

It's not too late. You can do it, and you can do a wonderful job at it. Entering medicine as a second career is increasingly common, and many medical schools are especially interested in applicants who have the maturity and skills that come from taking time to work and have other, "real-life" experiences rather than going straight from college to medical school. While students who are older can feel somewhat distanced from their younger peers, one of the keys to making this work is to seek out schools that enroll many nontraditional students and value the unique knowledge and perspectives that they bring.

This is a case in which the financial implications of undergoing medical training deserve extra consideration, as it will require sacrificing an income for the four years of medical school and then spending at least three years in residency—and possibly more in the cases of longer residencies or additional fellowship training—earning what could be a lower salary than you currently have.

Depending on the age of your children, the concerns about flexibility and childcare may not apply in quite the same way for someone planning to begin medical school with young children as for someone hoping to have children during school and training. However, while parenting during the early years of children's lives can be especially draining, your children will always need you regardless of their ages, and their needs - and the time and nature of what is required to meet those needs - will continually evolve.

Choosing to pursue medicine will certainly take away from time spent with your children and family. It can be very rewarding, though, to have the possibility of giving your children a better, more financially secure, future and by modeling for them—especially for young girls—dedication and hard work and the fact that they can be anything they want to be.

You're going to get older either way, and you have a choice about whether you spend that time doing something you love vs. spending it doing something else.

—OMDG (commenter), March 25, 2015

Do Single Moms Go into Medicine?

Yes, medical training and practice as a single mother is certainly doable, with many of the same considerations described above that go into planning for medicine as a career change. This is a scenario in which arranging for multiple sources of reliable childcare is essential, as is taking a careful look at the financial impact of pursuing medical school. You might look into completing your basic science prerequisites at a community college that offers evening classes so as to continue earning an income at your current job for as long as possible and to save on tuition costs for those courses.

Given the added challenges of navigating medical training as a single parent, it might make sense for you to take the time to consider other careers in healthcare as well [including working as a nurse practitioner (NP), physician assistant (PA), pharmacist, optometrist, nurse, or midwife, to name a few of the options] and evaluate whether any of these might appeal to you and allow you to fulfill your goals with a bit more flexibility along the way. (See the next section for more details.) But ultimately, if you are determined to become a physician and, knowing the sacrifices and complications that the pursuit of that dream can involve, have a plan to make it work, then go for it!

What Type of Degree Is Right for Me?

MD vs. DO

The question of whether to pursue an MD vs. a DO, and whether that choice will impact future experiences and opportunities, has no clear consensus. Some note that being a DO can impact your ability to get into residency and fellowship, especially in competitive fields, and that you will need to work harder in order to prove yourself, such as by earning higher test scores and presenting an overall more competitive application. Others worry that having a DO may lead to an applicant being denied the opportunity to interview regardless of their accomplishments.

While there is some consensus that less of a bias exists in primary care than in some sub-specialties, multiple recent graduates of DO schools report that they have experienced no biases whatsoever and feel equally well-trained and employable as their MD peers. Others enjoy having the ability to offer the added layer of osteopathic manipulative medicine (OMM) to their patients. They also cite examples of numerous DOs who have matched into strong programs in a variety of fields.

Physician vs. NP/PA

A career as an NP or PA can also be extremely rewarding. In general, they allow much greater flexibility than as a physician. This extends to a number of realms:

- *Financial*: Fewer years of school and no residency/fellowship allow you to join the workforce and start earning a higher salary earlier, with less debt in the form of student loans. While NPs and PAs tend to earn less than physicians, the salaries for all of these fields vary widely between specialties, practice settings, and geographic regions. Additionally, in some cases, coursework can be done part time, allowing you to continue earning an income while working toward your degree.

- *Flexibility in terms of schedule*: Many moms who are NPs or PAs cite the ability to be home for dinner most nights, drop their kids off at school, and attend performances or sports events as key elements in their career decision. They also tend to have more consistent schedule s in general.
- *Flexibility in career*: In many instances, midlevel providers can work in various different areas of medicine without completely retraining, whereas a major shift between fields as a physician would require additional years of residency or fellowship.

Many women who pursued an MD/DO degree feel that they likely would have chosen a different path had they known about NP and PA degrees while in college and caution others against enrolling in medical school (versus PA, NP, or other types of programs) unless they feel that it is absolutely necessary to reach their career goals or that they will always regret not having tried for a career as a physician. Others love being physicians and can't imagine following any other path. All commenters encourage anyone interested in pursuing a career in medicine to consider the multitude of options available, including NP, PA, midwifery, nursing, and pharmacy, and to talk to and shadow as many people as possible to get a real sense of what it is like to practice in each field.

> Start at the end. What do you want your days to look like? Think of what you want THE END GOAL to look like and talk to doctors and nurses alike to figure out how you get there the most efficiently.
>
> —*Mommabee, May 16, 2016*

> For any woman who is embarking on a medical career it's incredibly important to consider how one's choice of career will affect one's ability to parent in a way that works best for you.
>
> —*ZebraARNP, June 8, 2016*

How Do I Decide on a Specialty?

Many women express concern about specialty choice when they are still premed or early in their medical training. It's important to remember that, until you have done your clinical rotations, you most likely won't know for sure what you want to pursue. It takes time to figure out what you love, not to mention to gain exposure to the various specialties, sub-specialties, and settings in which they are practiced. What type of patient population do you hope to serve? What type of area (rural vs. urban, academic vs. community hospital) do you hope to practice in? As with the decisions of whether or not to pursue medicine and what degree makes the most sense for you, it can be helpful to start at the end (once you have seen many examples of what the various endpoints can look like) and work backward to determine what path or paths will help you get there.

Things to remember:

- It will be hard no matter what, especially during your years of training. Remember that phase of your career is temporary, and you ultimately will have at least some control over your schedule once you are finished, though it might involve different types of sacrifices (salary, geographic location, etc.).
- It is not uncommon to question your decision, even after you have chosen a specialty. When experiencing doubt, it's best to take time (often 6 months to a year) before making a decision or a major change to really evaluate how you are feeling and what factors are making you feel that way. This is especially important if you have recently had a big life event like having a baby or beginning a training program. And if, after taking that time to think, you are still unhappy, it's okay to change tracks or even quit. Medicine and your career certainly are not the only things that matters in life. Your needs and happiness are important, too!
- No matter what path you choose, there will be sacrifices, which make it especially important to find a field that truly interests you. There is no "easy" specialty, so while the relative flexibility of one field compared to another can certainly play a role in your choice, it should not be the sole factor on which you base your decision. Choosing solely based on lifestyle can lead to boredom and burnout over time.
- No specialty, job title, or practice setting will make you love every moment of every day. Every field and position will have downsides; what you need to determine is which one will bring you the most joy and fulfillment *most of the time*, while allowing you to care for yourself and your loved ones in the way that you want to *most of the time*. There is no perfect arrangement. But many women are able to be mothers and to practice medicine in a way that works for them.

I know happy OB's and sad ones. I know happy IMs and sad ones. I also know pathologists with major regrets, unlike me. I guess my own rant here is to say choose what you enjoy and try to make your lifestyle work. Paths are unpredictable and contingent on jobs available at the time, but you do have some control if you work hard and find the right practice.

—*Gizabeth Shyder, July 11, 2013*

Every specialty has paths that students are not aware of during medical school. This is another reason to choose based on the work and types of interactions that bring you the most satisfaction and meaning. Talk to attendings who you admire and find out why they chose their field, what they love about their jobs, and what they wish were different. Finally, know that you can always shift what you do as you progress in your career. For instance, you could take a leadership role that involves more administrative time if you feel you want to limit the more time-demanding clinical duties.

—*KC, July 14, 2013*

Moving Forward

It can be wonderful to be a mother in medicine. Having a life outside of medicine, and specifically being a mother, can make you a better doctor with even more skills to connect with, empathize with, and counsel your patients. Doing work that you love and that brings you fulfillment can make you better able to parent and to focus on spending quality time with your family, even when that time is limited. And doing your best to balance work and family can set a strong example for your children, showing them that with persistence and determination, they, too, can grow up to do something that they love.

> For all of us mothers in medicine, we definitely did not pick the easy route in life, but I feel lucky to be where I am.
>
> —*WimWop, June 8, 2015*

> Last night, after kindergarten registration, I stared at my worn out sleeping daughter and I was proud of this model of motherhood I have provided for her…. My residency baby – she made me a mother in medicine. She made me a better person, a better doctor – and every moment of this struggle feels very worth it right now.
>
> —*Cutter, August 5, 2016*

Motherhood and medicine will always be challenging endeavors, each in their own right and especially when combined. The demands and difficulties of each are dynamic and unique, and managing to do both requires more than a little bit of help along the way. Who better, then, to guide and lift one another up than other Mothers in Medicine?

> Mothers in medicine need to support each other and the hierarchy of medicine shouldn't get in the way. As mothers in medicine start to rise up in the ranks, we can create a culture that supports other mothers, especially those who are still in training or early in their career. For some of us, showing this support comes in the form of blogging and writing and working for policy change. But for many of us, support comes in a quieter form. It can be asking questions of how another mother in medicine is doing –whether she's feeling stressed or guilty or exhausted. It can be breaking down the hierarchies and treating each other not as students and residents and attendings but instead as adults who share a common thread.
>
> —*Doctor Professor Mom, November 12, 2015*

We're on call at all hours for our families and for our patients. Let us continue to be on call for one another as well.

Erratum to: Choosing Where and How to Work

Andrea Flory

Erratum to:
Chapter 5 in: K. Chretien (ed.), *Mothers in Medicine,*
https://doi.org/10.1007/978-3-319-68028-6_5

The chapter was inadvertently published with author's personal email and postal address. This has now been removed by this erratum.

The updated online version of this chapter can be found at
https://doi.org/10.1007/978-3-319-68028-6_5

A. Flory, MD (✉)
Washington, DC, USA
e-mail: alflory@gmail.com

Index

© Springer International Publishing AG 2018
K. Chretien (ed.), *Mothers in Medicine*,
https://doi.org/10.1007/978-3-319-68028-6

Printed in the United States
By Bookmasters